Loneline

Science and Practice

Loneliness

Science and Practice

Edited by

Dilip V. Jeste, M.D.

Tanya T. Nguyen, Ph.D.

Nancy J. Donovan, M.D.

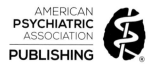

AMERICAN
PSYCHIATRIC
ASSOCIATION
PUBLISHING

If you wish to buy 50 or more copies of the same title, please go to www.appi.org/specialdiscounts for more information.

First Edition

Manufactured in the United States of America on acid-free paper
26   25   24   23   22   5   4   3   2   1

American Psychiatric Association Publishing
800 Maine Avenue SW, Suite 900
Washington, DC 20024-2812
www.appi.org

Library of Congress Cataloging-in-Publication Data
A CIP record is available from the Library of Congress.

British Library Cataloguing in Publication Data
A CIP record is available from the British Library.

Contents

Contributors

Manuela Barreto, Ph.D.
Professor of Social and Organizational Psychology, Department of Psychology, Washington Singer Laboratories, University of Exeter, Exeter, United Kingdom

Phaedra Bell, Ph.D.
Specialist, Department of Neurology, University of California San Francisco Weill Institute for Neurosciences; Senior Atlantic Fellow for Equity in Brain Health, University of California, San Francisco, San Francisco, California, and Trinity College, Dublin, Ireland

Susanne Buecker, Ph.D.
Professor, Department of Psychological Methods, Ruhr University Bochum, Bochum, Germany

Judith E. Carroll, Ph.D.
Associate Professor of Psychiatry and Biobehavioral Sciences, Cousins Center for Psychoneuroimmunology, Jane and Terry Semel Institute for Neuroscience and Human Behavior, University of California, Los Angeles, Los Angeles, California

Steve W. Cole, Ph.D.
Professor of Medicine and Psychiatry and Biobehavioral Sciences, Cousins Center for Psychoneuroimmunology, Jane and Terry Semel Institute for Neuroscience and Human Behavior, University of California, Los Angeles, Los Angeles, California

Yeates Conwell, M.D.
Professor, Department of Psychiatry, University of Rochester Medical Center, Rochester, New York

Nancy J. Donovan, M.D.
Chief, Division of Geriatric Psychiatry, Brigham and Women's Hospital; Associate Researcher, Massachusetts General Hospital; Associate Professor of Psychiatry, Harvard Medical School, Boston, Massachusetts

Alice Eccles, Ph.D.
Department of Psychology, University of Chester, Chester, United Kingdom

Miya M. Gentry, M.A.
Research Associate, Sam and Rose Stein Institute for Research on Aging, Department of Psychiatry, University of California San Diego, La Jolla, California

Louise Hawkley, Ph.D.
Principal Research Scientist, Academic Research Centers, National Opinion Research Center at the University of Chicago, Chicago Illinois

Julianne Holt-Lunstad, Ph.D.
Professor of Psychology and Neuroscience, Brigham Young University, Provo, Utah

Dilip V. Jeste, M.D.
Senior Associate Dean for Healthy Aging and Senior Care, Estelle and Edgar Levi Memorial Chair in Aging, Distinguished Professor of Psychiatry and Neurosciences, Director, Sam and Rose Stein Institute for Research on Aging, and Co-Director, IBM-UCSD Artificial Intelligence Center for Healthy Living, University of California San Diego, La Jolla, California

Dylan J. Jester, Ph.D., M.P.H.
Postdoctoral Fellow, Department of Psychiatry, Sam and Rose Stein Institute for Research on Aging, University of California San Diego, La Jolla, California

Jeffrey A. Lam, B.A.
Medical student, Warren Alpert Medical School, Brown University, Providence, Rhode Island

Brian Lawlor, M.D.
Conolly Norman Professor of Old Age Psychiatry, Trinity College; Deputy Executive Director, Global Brain Health Institute, University of California, San Francisco, San Francisco, California, and Trinity College, Dublin, Ireland

Ellen E. Lee, M.D.
Assistant Professor, Department of Psychiatry; Director, Division of Geriatric Psychiatry; and Faculty, Sam and Rose Stein Institute for Research on Aging, University of California San Diego; Staff Psychiatrist, Veterans Affairs San Diego Healthcare System, La Jolla, California

Maike Luhmann, Ph.D.
Professor, Department of Psychological Methods, Ruhr University Bochum, Bochum, Germany

Jürgen Margraf, Ph.D.
Professor, Mental Health Research and Treatment Center, Ruhr University Bochum, Bochum, Germany

Rio McLellan
Research Assistant, Department of Stem Cell Biology, Harvard University, Boston, Massachusetts

Tanya T. Nguyen, Ph.D.
Assistant Professor, Department of Psychiatry; Program Director, Senior Behavioral Health Intensive Outpatient Program; Sam and Rose Stein Institute for Research on Aging, University of California San Diego, La Jolla, California

Barton W. Palmer, Ph.D.
Staff Psychologist, Department of Mental Health, Veterans Affairs San Diego Healthcare System, San Diego; Professor, Department of Psychiatry, Sam and Rose Stein Institute for Research on Aging, University of California San Diego, LaJolla, California

Pamela Qualter, Ph.D.
Professor, Manchester Institute of Education, School of Environment, Education and Development, University of Manchester, Manchester, United Kingdom

Kelly E. Rentscher, Ph.D.
Assistant Professor of Psychiatry and Biobehavioral Sciences, Cousins Center for Psychoneuroimmunology, Jane and Terry Semel Institute for Neuroscience and Human Behavior, University of California, Los Angeles, Los Angeles, California

Lize Tibiriçá, Psy.D.
Postdoctoral Fellow, Department of Psychiatry, Stein Institute for Research on Aging, University of California San Diego, La Jolla, California

Kimberly A. Van Orden, Ph.D.
Associate Professor, Department of Psychiatry, University of Rochester Medical Center, Rochester, New York

Tilmann von Soest, Ph.D.
Professor in Psychology, PROMENTA Research Center, Department of Psychology, University of Oslo and Oslo Metropolitan University

Preface

INFORMED BY RESEARCH during the past half-century, the World Health Organization and other national health and health care bodies have increasingly emphasized the impact of social determinants of health on major health outcomes, including quality of life and longevity. One risk factor that has become increasingly prominent is loneliness—a subjective feeling of distress due to perceived social isolation. Loneliness has been shown to have major adverse mental and physical health effects throughout the life span. This book is, in part, a response to the National Academies of Science, Engineering and Medicine report released in early 2020 that called for screening for loneliness and social isolation in all health care practices and a need to develop best practices for addressing social isolation and loneliness in all medical subspecialty settings. This book was also motivated by our own observational research suggesting that certain cognitive and late-life developmental capacities, such as wisdom, may fortify against life experiences that predispose to loneliness. As the SARS-CoV-2 (COVID-19) pandemic and physical-distancing measures emerged in 2020, the need for the dissemination of knowledge of loneliness became even more pressing.

This book reviews the important and growing literature on loneliness, focusing on evidence-based findings. It addresses both the science and the everyday practice of mental health care that involves the psychobiology of loneliness, its appropriate clinical assessment, and strategies to prevent and manage its adverse consequences. The book has 10 chapters written by experts from North America and Europe. The first introductory chapter is followed by a chapter that presents the theoretical foundations of loneliness and other dimensions of social connection. The next three chapters discuss the epidemiology of loneliness during the life cycle and loneliness in specific populations, such as those with mental illnesses or members of marginalized communities. Chapters 6 and 7 are devoted to the neurobiological and systemic neuroendocrine and inflammatory mechanisms of loneliness. The last three chapters focus on interventions for loneliness: research-based interventions for younger and older age-groups and community-based interventions more broadly.

A book of this scope could not have been completed without the generosity and committed effort of our expert collaborators. We are deeply indebted to the contributing authors for sharing their leading expertise, for their many hours of preparation and writing, and for the excellence of their chapters. We are also grateful to American Psychiatric Association Publishing for their steady guidance before and during the process of developing this monograph. We particularly wish to acknowledge the encouragement and counsel provided by the editor-in-chief of our publisher, Laura Roberts, M.D. We also want to thank Paula Smith at UC San Diego, who provided administrative support for this project. Last, but not least, we are grateful for the support from our families whom we rely upon and love.

We hope this book will be a useful resource for clinicians, scientists, teachers, and administrators of health care systems and, most importantly, will contribute to the better mental and physical health of all people through greater understanding, prevention, and management of loneliness.

Dilip V. Jeste, M.D.

Tanya T. Nguyen, Ph.D.

Nancy J. Donovan, M.D.

1

Introduction

Tanya T. Nguyen, Ph.D.
Rio McLellan
Nancy J. Donovan, M.D.
Dilip V. Jeste, M.D.

Why Is Loneliness an Important Topic?

Human societies are changing rapidly. The ways we live, work, and connect with one another are evolving as we embrace increasingly digital methods of communication, changes in conventional education and employment practices, and the emergence of novel modes of social participation. While people are living longer, they are not necessarily experiencing parallel increases in quality of life, at least in recent years. The question remains: What contributes to living not just a longer but a better life? Over the past 80 years, the Harvard Study of Adult Development has sought to answer this question in the longest-standing longitudinal study on happiness. Since 1938, researchers have followed the lives of hundreds of individuals from adolescence, asking them regularly about their perceived quality of life (Mineo 2017). Intriguingly, they found that the number-one metric contributing to overall life satisfaction was not wealth, fame, or even general health but, rather, the maintenance of close personal relationships, which appears to reduce the risk of both physical and cognitive decline. These findings shed light on the critical importance of family, friendships, and community in shaping our lives and are a testament to the overall value of social relationships to humanity.

Human beings are fundamentally social creatures. Social interaction is correlated with increased survival rates for numerous species (McGlynn 2010). Social behavior originally evolved as an adaptive function to promote social bonding. Similar to other evolved aversive states, such as thirst, hunger, and pain, social isolation can evoke a negative subjective state to encourage fitness-enhancing behavior. A classic ecological example of how socialization acts as a protective mechanism is in its protection from predation. Social aggregation as protection has been documented extensively in the wild, from schools of fish to flocks of birds. Another driving mechanism behind the formation of social bonds is the potential for altruism and reciprocity—the "I help you, you help me" paradigm. Vampire bats are a model of such behavior; they share blood—their source of food—with other bats with whom they encounter and are likely to interact in the future (Wilkinson 1984). Essentially, these mutualistic relationships are formed with the hope that one bat's largesse today will be remembered in the future, and the favor will eventually be returned. Given that evolution is the active force underlying our drive for socialization, such altruistic interactions are rewarded in the form of overall health, well-being, and survival.

Increasingly over the past five decades, research on the social determinants of health, including education, occupation, income, inequality, racism and discrimination, working and living conditions, and food security, has begun to change our understanding of human health, disease, and well-being. The influence of social connections, both in terms of quantity and quality, is an important but often overlooked contributor to health outcomes. Two aspects of social relationships—loneliness and social isolation—have become increasingly prominent in the scientific literature as key constructs impacting human health. Individuals who are socially connected have been shown to have happier, healthier, and longer lives. In a study conducted by Berkman and Syme in 1979, the link between a metric quantifying social interactions and mortality was formalized. Their analysis demonstrated a twofold risk increase in relative mortality for the most socially isolated individuals in comparison with those who were socially integrated. In the years since the Berkman and Syme study, corroborative studies have amassed compelling evidence linking a lack of social connection to premature mortality. Biometric data, such as blood pressure, cholesterol, respiratory function, and electrocardiograms, support this association and revealed that subjects who reported higher levels of social relationships and activities were less likely to die during the follow-up periods (House et al. 1982; Orth-Gomér and Johnson 1987; Schoenbach et al. 1986; Welin et al. 1985). This research has considerable clinical relevance today, given that

24% of community-dwelling adults older than 65 years were categorized as being socially isolated in 2019, with 4% considered severely isolated (Cudjoe et al. 2020).

Current empirical research into loneliness and social isolation integrates broad, interdisciplinary scientific fields encompassing psychiatry, psychology, epidemiology, biology, and medicine. This has led to a number of terms being used (often interchangeably) to describe social relationships. Positive constructs include *social connection, social network, social integration,* and *social support,* and negative constructs include *social exclusion, social isolation, loneliness,* and *social deprivation.* However, as discussed in Chapter 2, "Loneliness, Other Aspects of Social Connection, and Their Measurement," there are important distinctions between these terms. *Social connection* is an overarching term that encompasses other commonly used terms. It is a multifactorial construct that describes the structural, functional, and quality aspects of human relationships and interactions (Donovan and Blazer 2020). Structural components entail the *existence of connections* among organized relationships and their roles. These tend to be inherently quantitative and therefore are relatively easy to evaluate, such as marital status or living arrangements. The functional aspects of relationships, on the other hand, are perceptual and thus can be more challenging to assess. These involve the *perceived functions* of relationships to individuals, such as received support or perceptions of loneliness. Even more difficult to measure, yet nevertheless important, are the qualities of these connections that reflect the degree of *positive* or *negative impact* that they have on a person's subjective well-being (Holt-Lunstad 2018).

Throughout this book, we primarily focus on the construct of loneliness. Although loneliness and social isolation are clearly related, it is important to distinguish between the two. *Loneliness* is the perception of social isolation or the subjective feeling of being socially disconnected, whereas *social isolation* is an objective lack or limited extent of social contacts with others. It is possible for a person to be socially isolated yet not experience loneliness, and vice versa. The common expression "lonely in a crowd" highlights this distinction and its variability among individuals. Although those who are socially isolated may feel lonely, loneliness and social isolation are often not highly correlated (Coyle and Dugan 2012), suggesting a need for development of differential or personalized treatment approaches.

Along with growing research identifying social isolation as a health risk, analogous studies have been performed in the context of loneliness. In the 1980s, sociobehavioral researchers codified the concept of loneliness and constructed a measuring system, the UCLA Loneliness Scale, which is still widely employed today (Russell 1996). Loneliness has been correlated with increased risk of mental illnesses, such as depression, anxiety, and suicidal ideation (Beutel et al. 2017), and with a 45% increased risk of death. Additionally, among those who report at least one symptom of loneliness, approximately 13% describe the symptom as occurring "often" (Perissinotto et al. 2012). Meta-analyses performed across many populations concerning loneliness have confirmed a 22%–26% increased likelihood of mortality as a result of loneliness (Holt-Lunstad et al. 2015; Rico-Uribe et al. 2018). As evidence mounts implicating loneliness as a predictor of disease and early death, urgency increases for the discovery and development of effective interventions.

The SARS-CoV-2 (COVID-19) pandemic beginning in March 2020 further exposed the importance of this issue and enhanced the need for effective and efficacious therapeutic interventions. Physical distancing precautions necessary to stem the spread of the virus dramatically altered the manner and frequency with which people interacted. A study in September 2020 confirmed a heightened prevalence of mental health, substance abuse, and suicidal ideation during the pandemic (Czeisler et al. 2021). This trade-off between risk and harm resulting from physical distancing has been described as the "social connectivity paradox"—the idea that activities that reduce risk of infection raise risk of loneliness (Smith et al. 2020). Thus, the global impact of COVID-19 has underscored the need for community-based and clinical interventions to combat loneliness and social isolation resulting from pandemic-related health precautions.

This book on the science and practice of loneliness aims to construct a translational framework for recognizing and addressing loneliness in a clinical context. We hope to provide a comprehensive summary of the current literature that is accessible and applicable to clinicians for identifying, diagnosing, and treating loneliness. In these chapters, we discuss how to assess loneliness, its epidemiology, its impacts on health outcomes, and the relevant research on interventions for different sociodemographic groups and in different contexts. With a coherent understanding of the incidence and distribution of loneliness and its various predictors and consequences, readers will develop the knowledge base necessary to combat this behavioral pandemic (Jeste et al. 2020).

Summary of Chapters

Chapter 2, by Donovan and Holt-Lunstad, presents original descriptions of loneliness by Weiss, Perlman and Peplau, and others that provide a theoretical foundation for our understanding of loneliness that is enduring and compassionate in nature. Loneliness is viewed as a form of social and psychological distress corresponding to basic human needs for intimate connection (emotional loneliness), sustaining social relations (social loneliness), and collective engagement with others (collective loneliness). There is a genetically based natural variation in the susceptibility to loneliness among people that can be seen as adaptive to societies as a whole. Experiences of loneliness and its subtypes are also influenced by developmental experiences, psychological attributions, culture, life stage, and changes in the availability of social relationships. Mental health practitioners are well-positioned to recognize these individual differences and contributing factors and their implications for selecting personalized, therapeutic approaches and interventions. Loneliness is also discussed as a specific component of the broader construct of social connection that the describes structural, functional, and quality aspects of human relationships and interactions. Measurement approaches to loneliness and other aspects of social connection are reviewed, and representative measures relevant to clinical use are provided and referenced in the chapter appendix.

In Chapter 3, "Loneliness Across the Life Span," Luhmann and colleagues show that, despite being a relatively stable construct, loneliness can and does change across the life span. Some cross-sectional and longitudinal studies indicate that loneliness may decrease during childhood and adolescence and increase in old age, particularly after age 80. Age differences in loneliness can be explained by age differences in the prevalence of relevant risk factors. Older people are particularly at higher risk of feeling lonely because widowhood, social isolation, and functional limitations due to poor health are more common in this age group. With aging, the *quantity* of one's social relationships becomes less important than the *quality* of those relationships; therefore, age-appropriate strategies should employed to identify and reach lonely people. Younger people are more likely than older adults to benefit from interventions aimed at establishing opportunities for social interactions and improving positive social engagement.

Gentry and Palmer, in Chapter 4 ("Loneliness in People Living With Mental Health Disorders"), differentiate acute and chronic loneliness. *Acute* loneliness is thought to be an adaptive motivator for social connection, but when loneliness becomes *chronic*, it can trigger a self-defeating set of problems arising from distorted perceptions of self and others and can be associated with heightened arousal that may lead to adverse health outcomes. The adverse health outcomes associated with disorders such as schizophrenia and PTSD overlap with those associated with loneliness, but the temporal associations of such relationships and points of intervention remain unclear. Studies concerning the prevalence of loneliness in those with schizophrenia have increased in recent years, reporting remarkably high rates of 43%–80%. Loneliness and depression are separate constructs despite their frequent co-occurrence and bidirectional impacts. Loneliness and anxiety also influence each other and frequently co-occur. There is less literature on the interaction of loneliness and bipolar disorder or PTSD, signaling a need for further empirical research in these areas. Response to solitude (being alone) varies across individuals and sometimes within the same individual at different times. A person may desire connection yet feel fear or hopeless about such connection. Some may find it difficult to tolerate solitude because they experience distorted thoughts about what it means to be alone, whereas others may associate positive solitude with a sense of greater well-being. These are all points of potential intervention, and clinicians should work in partnership with each patient to identify possible causes and manage them.

Chapter 5 ("Loneliness in Marginalized Communities"), by Tibiriçá and colleagues, discusses loneliness in marginalized communities such as people from racial and ethnic minorities, those who are LGBTQ+, and immigrants. It presents an overview, based on empirical literature, of the impact of culture and discrimination/marginalization on the prevalence and experience of loneliness, on risk and protective factors, and downstream on health, well-being, and mortality. Much of the research from North America on loneliness has focused on samples predominantly comprising cisgender, heterosexual, non-Latinx white adults. Yet there are strong reasons to suspect that experiences of marginalization, bigotry, and discrimination affect subjective and objective aspects of social isolation; we cannot generalize findings from loneliness research on relatively homogeneous, nonmarginalized persons to those in various marginalized groups. Loneliness is common among marginalized communities, although prevalence figures vary across studies. More research is needed to address inconsistent findings from different studies, which may be due to the use of different measures, over- versus underreporting of symptoms, and varied levels of underrepresentation of different races/ethnicities. These groups also commonly face health and health care inequities, and clinicians must focus on ensuring patients' access to necessary community resources. Future studies should also examine intragroup racial/ethnic variations in loneliness in order to understand heterogeneity among groups. This is especially true for Hispanic/Latinx groups in the United States. Much of the work thus far has entirely disregarded the within-group heterogeneity masked by the label of Hispanic/Latinx ethnicity, failing to discern any differences between individuals of Mexican, Puerto Rican, Central American, and Cuban ethnicity, all of whom have unique immigration, discrimination, and acculturation experiences in the United States. As the U.S. population demographics shift, with current racial/ethnic minority groups becoming the majority, referring to white people as the uniform reference group may need to be qualified. Finally, published results usually reflect cross-sectional data, thus limiting analysis and interpretation regarding causality. Self-report has its own set of limitations as well. Longitudinal investigations using some objective measures are clearly needed.

In Chapter 6, Lam and Lee discuss the "Neurobiology of Loneliness." Based on a review of brain imaging studies using CT, MRI, functional MRI, diffusion tensor imaging (DTI), SPECT, and PET, as well as electroencephalography and postmortem brain tissue analysis, they find strong evidence that loneliness is associated with differences in social brain regions, including the parts responsible for mental representations of self and the affective, perceptual, and attentional systems. Loneliness has been associated with abnormal structure or function of the prefrontal cortex, insula, and ventral striatum and physiologically with the default mode, attentional, and visual networks. Loneliness also has a strong relationship with dementia, specifically Alzheimer's disease. Collectively, the current literature provides evidence that loneliness may increase hypervigilance and alter social approach motivation, which supports the theory that loneliness evolved as a means to increase reproductive fitness. Future studies should examine the impact of loneliness interventions on brain function to better understand the underlying mechanisms of social functioning.

Loneliness is associated with the activation of several neuroendocrine and inflammatory pathways that may be adaptive for short-term survival but detrimental for long-term health, increasing risk for morbidity and early mortality. In Chapter 7, "Systemic Neuroendocrine and Inflammatory Mechanisms in Loneliness," Rentscher and colleagues comment on one general pathway through which loneliness may be associated with worsening health, involving CNS-mediated alterations in neural and endocrine activity. This can subsequently affect immune function in ways that may both promote the development and progression of chronic disease and reciprocally feed back to the brain to amplify and prolong experiences of social threat and loneliness. Loneliness may influence leukocyte composition through sympathetic innervation of the bone marrow, increasing immature monocytes in circulation and contributing to systemic inflammation. Loneliness is also associated with a higher cortisol awakening response (CAR) in young and middle-aged adults but a lower CAR in older adults, which may have detrimental effects on health, including greater wear and tear and poorer inflammatory regulation by cortisol. Loneliness is associated with increased proinflammatory gene expression and decreased glucocorticoid receptor and antiviral gene expression and transcription control pathways. Inflammation can reciprocally influence perceptions of threat and social withdrawal, driving further loneliness. Intervening to stop this feedforward loop is critical for public health. Studies show that stress-reducing practices of mindfulness and meditation downregulate loneliness-related proinflammatory gene expression, further supporting the association between the neurobiology of loneliness and immune response (Black and Slavich 2016; Creswell et al. 2012).

In Chapter 8, Qualter and colleagues address "Interventions for Loneliness in Younger People." Loneliness among children and adolescents is associated with depression, social anxiety, self-harm, worse self-reported health and sleep, low academic performance, and struggles in employment. Risk factors for youth loneliness span individual, interpersonal, situational, and sociocultural levels. The evaluated interventions focus primarily on individual differences and interpersonal and situational risk factors, targeting social and emotional skills development, social isolation, and social support. Only a small number of interventions have been shown to be successful at reducing youth loneliness. The most successful are psychological therapies, including emotional/social skill development, adaptive coping mechanisms, enhancement of social support, and increasing peer interaction. The focus of such interventions is on managing the maladaptive cognitions associated with loneliness and adopting adaptive coping strategies. However, interventions that address the sociocultural factors linked to youth loneliness are lacking. Tackling loneliness goes beyond the individual and their immediate relationships, with interventions needing to recognize and address other aspects of the systems in which social relationships take place.

Chapter 9, by Van Orden and Conwell, reviews "Interventions for Loneliness in Older Adults." With advancing age, older adults are at increasing risk for loneliness because they are more likely to live alone, experience the loss of loved ones, endure negative mental and physical health outcomes, and lack social support for emotional well-being (National Academies of Sciences, Engineering, and Medicine 2020). Individualized prevention and treatment for loneliness in older adults should begin with analysis of the pathways contributing to the person's social disconnections. Loneliness is modifiable. Behavioral interventions can reduce loneliness and social isolation for older adults, but it is not clear yet which interventions are most effective, for whom, or in what circumstances nor is it clear what mechanisms are essential to achieve positive outcomes. Some evidence indicates that loneliness brought on by mental health issues may be ameliorated through psychotherapy or mindfulness training, whereas loneliness caused by sensory limitations and physical disorders might be better targeted through appropriate health care, wellness, and exercise classes. Community-based programs that address loneliness in older adults include AARP's Connect2Affect (https://connect2affect.org) resource list and the United Kingdom's Campaign to End Loneliness (www.campaigntoendloneliness.org). Some programs for loneliness may not be acceptable to older adults, necessitating research codesign and the involvement of older adults in all phases of research. The COVID-19 pandemic highlighted the importance of understanding whether interventions for social connection are effective when delivered via videocall or online. Future work should continue to investigate the advantages and disadvantages of remote versus in-person modes of delivery for programs to address loneliness.

Chapter 10, by Bell and Lawlor, describes "Community-Based Interventions for Loneliness." Because the causes of loneliness are often structural and socially determined, the informed design of a more connected, prosocial society is highly promising for decreasing loneliness on a larger scale. Different strategies of execution exist for community-based mediation, including preventive and interventional approaches. Preventive techniques are steps toward preempting the development of loneliness in the general population and in individuals at elevated risk, whereas interventional techniques are aimed at those already experiencing loneliness. Primary prevention measures begin early in schools to increase awareness of the importance of social connection for health in order to short circuit the development of chronic loneliness in at-risk children and adolescents. Primary prevention approaches also involve increasing access to available community activities. Secondary and tertiary interventions offer more individualized treatment and cater to high-risk persons or those who are lonely. Various strategies within this framework include *social prescribing*— the connection of formal health care systems and local community organizations, peer befriendings, virtual/digital support, and intergenerational programs. In light of the COVID-19 pandemic, it is also important to acknowledge remotely delivered community interventions via phone and video call. In addition to cost-effective community interventions, multileveled public policies that prioritize social health within populations are also needed. Governments should address and prioritize the short- and long-term effects of loneliness and social isolation on health and quality of life. Greater attention must be paid to the evaluation and design of the built environment, social spaces, and social services to decrease loneliness and isolation as a matter of public policy and across sectors at the community level. Methodologically strong research is needed for establishing a comprehensive evidence base to inform effective public policies and community interventions for loneliness.

Emerging Trends

One book alone cannot cover the entire field of science and practice in a fast-growing area of research interest and public health significance such as loneliness. Loneliness is a complex, multifaceted condition emerging from sociocultural, biological, and personal contexts. Although loneliness is a part of human nature, data suggest a marked increase in its prevalence and in associated conditions, such as suicides and substance abuse, in recent decades. The Centers for Disease Control and Prevention reported a 33% increase in suicides and sixfold increase in opioid-related deaths in the United States from 1999 to 2017. Moreover, loneliness has not only impacted the health and longevity of individuals but also of businesses and governments, which have recognized financial losses because of loneliness among workers. At least two countries, the United Kingdom and Japan, have appointed new "ministers of loneliness." It seems that a silent behavioral pandemic of loneliness had been developing for more than two decades preceding the COVID-19 pandemic (Jeste et al. 2020). Although loneliness remains a difficult problem to tackle, new research is being conducted each year, offering hope of identifying effective interventions.

Sometimes, surprising findings emerge that reveal new avenues of investigation. For example, during the COVID-19 pandemic, it was widely expected that older adults would experience more psychological harm than younger adults because of their higher risk of physical complications and mortality and the barriers they face in accessing technology that allows social communication despite physical distancing. Yet multiple studies across the world have shown *lower* prevalence rates of mental and behavioral health symptoms among older compared with younger adults, differences attributed to older adults' higher levels of resilience, compassion, and wisdom (Vahia et al. 2020). A survey of 945 Americans ages 18–76 years showed that older age was associated with higher frequency and intensity of positive emotions and lower frequency and intensity of negative emotions (Carstensen et al. 2020). Another survey of 5,186 U.S. adults reported age-related differences in rates of mental health symptoms (e.g., anxiety, depression, perceived stress): 15% in adults older than 65 and 75% in those ages 18–24 (Czeisler et al. 2021). Interviews among older adults have elucidated commonly used coping strategies to combat loneliness, including acceptance of aging, compassion, spirituality, seeking companionship, community environments, and "oneliness"—comfort in being alone (Morlett Paredes et al. 2021). Notably, several of these coping strategies (i.e., acceptance of aging, compassion, and spirituality) align with the components of wisdom.

Wisdom is a holistic, multidimensional trait comprising prosocial behaviors, emotional regulation, self-reflection, spirituality, acceptance of divergent values, decisiveness, and social advising (Jeste and Lee 2019). Importantly, there is a strong inverse relationship between loneliness and wisdom that has been replicated in multiple independent samples, from a community-dwelling cohort in San Diego, California (Jeste et al. 2021; Lee et al. 2019) to a nationwide cohort recruited via Web survey (Nguyen et al. 2020) and a cross-cultural cohort of middle-age and oldest-old adults (including nonagenarians) in Cilento, Italy (Jeste et al. 2021; Lee et al. 2019). Even biological (electroencephalography and microbiome) and longitudinal clinical studies support the inverse relationship between loneliness and wisdom (Grennan et al. 2021; Lee et al. 2019; Nguyen et al. 2021). These findings suggest that wisdom may be protective against loneliness and that interventions that enhance wisdom may also ameliorate loneliness.

Of the different components of wisdom, prosocial behaviors, which include empathy, compassion, and altruism, are most strongly related to loneliness and therefore may be a heuristic framework for clinical interventions. We can anticipate the development and testing of new interventions of this type in the coming years.

With this book we hope to give readers the information and tools required to address loneliness in a clinical setting. By covering the existing literature and exploring a variety of assessment and interventional strategies, it will hopefully serve as a guide for addressing the negative health outcomes of loneliness at personal and societal levels and for promoting well-being in individuals and societies as a whole.

Suggested Readings

Cacioppo JT, Cacioppo S: Loneliness in the modern age: an evolutionary theory of loneliness (ETL). Adv Exp Soc Psychol 58:127–197, 2018

Cacioppo JT, Hawkley LC, Thisted RA: Perceived social isolation makes me sad: 5-year cross-lagged analyses of loneliness and depressive symptomatology in the Chicago Health, Aging, and Social Relations Study. Psychol Aging 25(2):453–463, 2010 20545429

DiJulio B, Hamel L, Muñana C, Brodie M: Loneliness and social isolation in the United States, the United Kingdom, and Japan: an international survey. Oakland, CA, Kaiser Family Foundation, August 30, 2018

Donovan NJ, Blazer D: Social isolation and loneliness in older adults: review and commentary of a National Academies Report. Am J Geriatr Psychiatry 28(12):1233–1244, 2020 32919873

Jeste DV, Lee EE: The emerging empirical science of wisdom: definition, measurement, neurobiology, longevity, and interventions. Harv Rev Psychiatry 27(3):127–140, 2019 31082991

References

Berkman LF, Syme SL: Social networks, host resistance, and mortality: a nine-year follow-up study of Alameda County residents. Am J Epidemiol 109(2):186–204, 1979 425958

Beutel ME, Klein EM, Brähler E, et al: Loneliness in the general population: prevalence, determinants and relations to mental health. BMC Psychiatry 17(1):97, 2017 28320380

Black DS, Slavich GM: Mindfulness meditation and the immune system: a systematic review of randomized controlled trials. Ann N Y Acad Sci 1373(1):13–24, 2016 26799456

Carstensen LL, Shavit YZ, Barnes JT: Age advantages in emotional experience persist even under threat from the COVID-19 pandemic. Psychol Sci 31(11):1374-1385, 2020 33104409

Coyle CE, Dugan E: Social isolation, loneliness and health among older adults. J Aging Health 24(8):1346–1363, 2012 23006425

Creswell JD, Irwin MR, Burklund LJ, et al: Mindfulness-based stress reduction training reduces loneliness and pro-inflammatory gene expression in older adults: a small randomized controlled trial. Brain Behav Immun 26(7):1095–1101, 2012 22820409

Cudjoe TKM, Roth DL, Szanton SL, et al: The epidemiology of social isolation: National Health and Aging Trends Study. J Gerontol B Psychol Sci Soc Sci 75(1):107–113, 2020 29590462

Czeisler MÉ, Lane RI, Wiley JF, et al: Follow-up survey of US adult reports of mental health, substance use, and suicidal ideation during the COVID-19 pandemic, September 2020. JAMA Netw Open 4(2):e2037665, 2021 33606030

Donovan NJ, Blazer D: Social isolation and loneliness in older adults: review and commentary of a National Academies Report. Am J Geriatr Psychiatry 28(12):1233–1244, 2020 32919873

Grennan G, Balasubramani PP, Alim F, et al: Cognitive and neural correlates of loneliness and wisdom during emotional bias. Cereb Cortex 31(7):3311–3322, 2021

Holt-Lunstad J: Why social relationships are important for physical health: a systems approach to understanding and modifying risk and protection. Annu Rev Psychol 69(Jan):437–458, 2018 29035688

Holt-Lunstad J, Smith TB, Baker M, et al: Loneliness and social isolation as risk factors for mortality: a meta-analytic review. Perspect Psychol Sci 10(2):227–237, 2015 25910392

House JS, Robbins C, Metzner HL: The association of social relationships and activities with mortality: prospective evidence from the Tecumseh Community Health Study. Am J Epidemiol 116(1):123–140, 1982 7102648

Jeste DV, Lee EE: The emerging empirical science of wisdom: definition, measurement, neurobiology, longevity, and interventions. Harv Rev Psychiatry 27(3):127–140, 2019 31082991

Jeste DV, Lee EE, Cacioppo S: Battling the modern behavioral epidemic of loneliness: suggestions for research and interventions. JAMA Psychiatry 77(6):553–554, 2020 32129811

Jeste DV, Di Somma S, Lee EE, et al: Study of loneliness and wisdom in 482 middle-aged and oldest-old adults: a comparison between people in Cilento, Italy and San Diego, USA. Aging Ment Health 25(11):2149–2159, 2021 33000647

Lee EE, Depp C, Palmer BW, et al: High prevalence and adverse health effects of loneliness in community-dwelling adults across the lifespan: role of wisdom as a protective factor. Int Psychogeriatr 31(10):1447–1462, 2019 30560747

McGlynn T: How does social behavior evolve? Nature Education Knowledge 1(8):33, 2010

Mineo L: Good genes are nice, but joy is better. The Harvard Gazette, April 11, 2017

Morlett Paredes A, Lee EE, Chik L, et al: Qualitative study of loneliness in a senior housing community: the importance of wisdom and other coping strategies. Aging Ment Health 25(3):559–566, 2021 31918561

National Academies of Sciences, Engineering, and Medicine: Social Isolation and Loneliness in Older Adults: Opportunities for the Health Care System. Washington, DC, National Academies Press, 2020

Nguyen TT, Lee EE, Daly RE, et al: Predictors of loneliness by age decade: study of psychological and environmental factors in 2,843 community-dwelling Americans aged 20–69 years. J Clin Psychiatry 81(6):20m13378, 2020 33176072

Nguyen TT, Zhang X, Wu TC, et al: Association of loneliness and wisdom with gut microbial diversity and composition: an exploratory study. Front Psychiatry 12:648475, 2021

Orth-Gomér K, Johnson JV: Social network interaction and mortality: a six year follow-up study of a random sample of the Swedish population. J Chronic Dis 40(10):949–957, 1987 3611293

Perissinotto CM, Stijacic Cenzer I, Covinsky KE: Loneliness in older persons: a predictor of functional decline and death. Arch Intern Med 172(14):1078–1083, 2012 22710744

Rico-Uribe LA, Caballero FF, Martín-María N, et al: Association of loneliness with all-cause mortality: a meta-analysis. PLoS One 13(1):e0190033, 2018 29300743

Russell DW: UCLA Loneliness Scale (Version 3): reliability, validity, and factor structure. J Pers Assess 66(1):20–40, 1996 8576833

Schoenbach VJ, Kaplan BH, Fredman L, Kleinbaum DG: Social ties and mortality in Evans County, Georgia. Am J Epidemiol 123(4):577–591, 1986 3953538

Smith ML, Steinman LE, Casey EA: Combatting social isolation among older adults in a time of physical distancing: the COVID-19 social connectivity paradox. Front Public Health 8(July):403, 2020 32850605

Vahia IV, Jeste DV, Reynolds CF III: Older adults and the mental health effects of COVID-19. JAMA 324(22):2253–2254, 2020 33216114

Welin L, Tibblin G, Svärdsudd K, et al: Prospective study of social influences on mortality: the study of men born in 1913 and 1923. Lancet 1(8434):915–918, 1985 2858755

Wilkinson GS: Reciprocal food sharing in the vampire bat. Nature 308(5955):181–184, 1984

2

Loneliness, Other Aspects of Social Connection, and Their Measurement

Nancy J. Donovan, M.D.
Julianne Holt-Lunstad, Ph.D.

> One of the burdens of loneliness is that we have so many
> preconceptions regarding its nature, so many defenses against
> recognizing its pain, and so little knowledge of how to help.
>
> *Frieda Fromm-Reichmann (1959)*

The authors would like to thank Kelsey Biddle for her assistance in the preparation
of the chapter.

WRITING OF LONELINESS IN 1959, Frieda Fromm-Reichmann noted "a strange reluctance on the part of psychiatrists to seek scientific clarification of the subject. Thus, it comes about that loneliness is one of the least satisfactorily conceptualized psychological phenomena, not even mentioned in most psychiatric textbooks" (Fromm-Reichmann 1959, p. 1). She and, later, other loneliness researchers attributed this avoidance to the anxiety that loneliness elicits in others and a common response to marginalize those who are lonely. "Loneliness seems to be such a painful, frightening experience that people will do practically everything to avoid it" (p. 1). The goal of this chapter is to provide a clinically meaningful picture of loneliness so that it can be recognized and understood in patients presenting for mental health care.

In this chapter, we present complementary perspectives on the nature of loneliness from the past 50 years. We begin with a summary of early academic literature, which described loneliness as a state of social and psychological distress corresponding to the basic human needs for intimate connection, sustaining social relations, and collective engagement with others. Genetic influences have been characterized more recently, providing a fuller understanding of genetic, developmental, psychological, social, and life-phase impacts on loneliness.

Because loneliness is central to human mental and physical health, there is a pressing need to develop standardized and validated approaches and tools for its assessment and that of other forms of social disconnection within health care practices and systems, including mental health care. To that end, we also present a larger view of *social connection*, a term that encompasses multiple aspects of relationship quantity, quality, and function. This provides a framework for understanding how the subjective experience of loneliness relates to objective, quantitative deficits in social ties (*social isolation*) or other provisions of social relationships (*social support*). Identifying the precise area of social disconnection is critical to selecting an effective intervention or approach to care. In later sections of this chapter, we discuss validated rating scales developed in research studies and the clinical assessment of loneliness and other forms of social disconnection.

Social and Psychological Contributions to Loneliness

In 1973, sociologist Robert Weiss brought new attention to the phenomena of loneliness in his book *Loneliness: The Experience of Emotional and Social Isolation* (Weiss 1973). Nearly five decades later, his fundamental description of loneliness holds true. He wrote, "Loneliness is not caused by being alone but by being without some definite needed relationship or set of relationships" such as an "intimate attachment," "meaningful friendships," or "other linkages to a coherent community" (p. 17). In describing loneliness as a "response to a relational deficit" he noted that these "different forms of loneliness are responsive to different remedies" (p. 18). Weiss and colleagues such as John Bowlby discussed the nature and development of affectional bonds during the life course and their vulnerability to disruption. Experiences of loneliness are often linked to developmental stages, life circumstances, and life events. In Weiss's view, "ordinary loneliness" encompasses two main components: the loneliness of *emotional isolation* and the loneliness of *social isolation*.

Emotional loneliness is seen as derived from the lifelong need for a "primary, security-providing attachment" that begins with the mother–infant bond (Weiss 1973, p. 93). In later stages of life, this attachment is often characterized by companionate love, compassion, understanding, sexual desire, the giving and receiving of love, the sharing of work, and other life experiences. Physical proximity or cohabiting also characterizes this form of attachment. Disruption of this attachment can lead to sudden emotional loneliness and be experienced as anxiety, restlessness, apprehension, or emptiness.

According to Weiss, the benefits of broader social relationships are distinct from those of attachment, and these provisions do not substitute for each other. Distress due to social isolation or exclusion from peers appears early in childhood. Engagement with peers, social participation, and social acceptance become increasingly important during childhood and adolescence and facilitate the formation of self-identity during adolescence. In adulthood, social networks provide a base for social activities, sources of information, help with decision-making, and tangible forms of support. Compared with emotional loneliness, *social loneliness* is less likely to occur suddenly except in certain contexts, such as a geographical move. Although both forms of loneliness are linked to dissatisfaction and depression, in Weiss's formulation social loneliness is dominated by boredom and aimlessness and feelings of marginality rather than the anxiety and apprehension of emotional isolation.

Daniel Perlman and Letitia Peplau further described the nature of human loneliness in 1981, emphasizing its subjective quality and psychological influences (Perlman and Peplau 1981). They conceptualized loneliness as the discrepancy between one's desired and achieved levels of social relations, sometimes called the "discrepancy, attributional approach to loneliness" (Perlman and Peplau 1981, p. 32). This occurs when "social relations are deficient in some important way, either quantitatively or qualitatively"

(p. 31). Loneliness is aversive, an unpleasant and emotionally intense experience, a feeling of alienation.

Like Weiss and earlier theorists, Perlman and Peplau distinguished this dysphoric form of loneliness from other states. *Existential loneliness*, an alternate form of loneliness, is an experience of human self-confrontation and growth that has both positive and negative attributes. (Moustakas 1961). Perlman and Peplau (1981) also referenced an apathetic form of loneliness in which lonely individuals are accepting or resigned to their condition and no longer distressed. Thus, these researchers built on the work of Weiss to examine the experiences and "normal ranges of loneliness among the general public" (p. 32) that are subjective in nature but arise from the structure and dynamics of human relationships.

Perlman and Peplau described a large array of "antecedent" factors that predispose individuals to loneliness, even if they are not the immediate cause (Table 2–1). Cognitive processes interact with these antecedent factors, giving rise to loneliness in some but not all individuals. Cognitive processes are a function of culture, language, and individual differences, including differing attributions to loneliness. Attributions can influence loneliness persistence and severity, for instance, the attribution of loneliness to failure or to being unattractive. Other attributions include a sense of lacking control over loneliness or overestimating the uniqueness of one's situation. Prevailing attitudes and biases about loneliness on the part of others can also influence the course of loneliness. Lonely individuals are often avoided or rejected and can be viewed as justifiably rejected or intentionally reclusive. It has also been proposed that those who recognize loneliness in others may fear being similarly ostracized or lonely. Individuals with low social status or who differ from group norms are most adversely affected by these biases. Importantly, certain cognitive and behavioral manifestations of loneliness can also perpetuate it, such as increased anxiety and vigilance about interpersonal relationships and avoidance of social interactions due to a biased expectation of negative reactions from others.

Contemporaneous with this work, Dan Russell and colleagues developed the UCLA Loneliness Scale (UCLA LS), which defined a psychometrically valid loneliness construct with a unidimensional structure (Russell 1996; Russell et al. 1978, 1980). This development was a major step toward detecting and measuring loneliness—as advanced by Weiss, Perlman and Peplau, and others—at a population level. The De Jong Gierveld Scale was also developed and validated to measure loneliness as a single entity with two subcomponents corresponding to emotional loneliness and social loneliness (De Jong Gierveld 1987; De Jong Gierveld and Van Tilburg 2006) (see chapter appendix).

TABLE 2-1.   Antecedents of loneliness as described by Perlman and Peplau (1981)

Categories	Types	Examples
Changes in achieved social relations	Termination	Widowhood
	Physical separation	Moving, summer camp, university
	Status change	Retirement, unemployment, new parenthood
Changes in desired social relations	Developmental changes	Need for intimacy beginning in preadolescence, greater emphasis on social relations in mid- to late life
	Situational changes	Holidays, periods of stress
	Changes in expectations	Increased expectations during illness or transitions
Quantity and quality of social contacts	Quantity	Dating less, fewer social activities, more interactions with casual acquaintances or strangers than with close friends
	Quality	Marital dissatisfaction, less rewarding relationships
Personal factors	Shyness	Avoidance of social interactions, less initiative in conversations
	Self-esteem	Self-blame for loneliness
	Social skills	Problems making friends, introducing oneself, making phone calls; different style of interacting; self-focused, nonresponsive
	Similarity	Different personal characteristics from group norm
	Demographic characteristics	Being unmarried, lower socio-economic status, age (late adolescence)
	Childhood antecedents	Parental divorce, remote parenting style and lack of warmth or support, parental rejection

TABLE 2–1.   **Antecedents of loneliness as described by Perlman and Peplau (1981) *(continued)***

Categories	Types	Examples
Cultural and situational factors	Cultural values	Emphasis on independence, competition vs. community, mutual dependence
	Social norms	Expected time frame for dating and marriage
	Cultural expectations	Being alone on Saturday night
	Situational constraints	Built environment, architecture of housing affecting socialization

Others have studied the psychometric properties of these loneliness scales to explore components within the main loneliness construct. Using the 20-item version of the UCLA LS (Russell et al. 1980), Hawkley et al. (2005) identified three distinct underlying components (related clusters of items), classified as *isolation*, *relational connectedness*, and *collective connectedness* in both younger and older age samples. Quantitative ratings of three types of social relationship (i.e., marriage/partnership, friends/family, and group participation) were analyzed as predictors of these loneliness components. Isolation, which corresponds to feelings of pervasive aloneness and rejection, was most strongly and negatively predicted by marriage or living with a partner. Relational connectedness, which corresponds to feelings of familiarity, closeness, and support, was most strongly predicted by numbers of friends and relatives. Collective connectedness, which corresponds to group identification and cohesion, was most strongly predicted by group membership. Thus, the third component of the UCLA LS provided evidence for a distinct form of loneliness related to group or collective identity—in addition to emotional and social loneliness—that has been recognized but less emphasized in the loneliness literature.

Genetic Contributions to Loneliness

Other theorists have articulated the importance of loneliness to the survival of individuals and groups and the natural variation in susceptibility to loneliness within a population. Rather than considering loneliness an aberrant psychosocial state, it is seen as a conserved biological response. Both genes and social environment contribute to the experience of loneliness.

The evolutionary theory of loneliness holds that it is an innate response that signals when important social relations are endangered or damaged and prompts the person to reconnect with others (Cacioppo et al. 2014). Behavioral and biological responses to loneliness serve to increase motivation to approach others and to alter social behavior to avoid negative events (Spithoven et al. 2019).

Research in behavioral genetics has found that genetic factors account for 0.37–0.55 of the variance for loneliness in the population (Spithoven et al. 2019). Genetic factors are understood to influence a person's susceptibility to loneliness in different social conditions or environments. Thus, *susceptibility* to loneliness, not level of loneliness, may be inherited. Many genes contribute in small degree to this overall susceptibility and show coheritability with certain personality characteristics, such as neuroticism and, negatively and less strongly, extraversion (Gao et al. 2017). These genetic factors have more complex coheritability patterns with major psychiatric conditions, such as depression and schizophrenia (Gao et al. 2017). Therefore, the expression of loneliness in the pathogenesis of these mental health disorders may relate to the shared environmental influences and the effects of loneliness interacting with psychiatric symptoms. Notably, the nature and strength of these associations may vary across the life span (Abdellaoui et al. 2018; Qualter et al. 2015).

The variability in loneliness as a trait and the behavioral diversity it implies are proposed to be adaptive at a population level. For example, some group members are more exploratory and less prone to loneliness and therefore provide specific benefits to the group, such as acquired knowledge from the outside world (Cacioppo and Cacioppo 2012). More closely embedded members may be more sensitive to separation from others and provide different, stable benefits, such as nurturance and protection of the group (Cacioppo and Cacioppo 2012). In this way, varying susceptibilities to loneliness are understood to confer a range of benefits for the prosperity and survival of human societies.

Figure 2–1 shows a conceptual representation of the interaction between a single gene (genotype) and the environment that gives rise to a "reaction norm," or the strength of a behavioral outcome such as loneliness, in different environmental conditions (Spithoven et al. 2019). Certain genotypes show an enhanced behavioral response to environmental stimuli that trigger loneliness. The behavioral and physiological responses of loneliness are thought to be driven by epigenetic processes such as DNA methylation and histone methylation and acetylation in the brain regions involved in stress physiology and social emotional and behavioral processes (Spithoven et al. 2019).

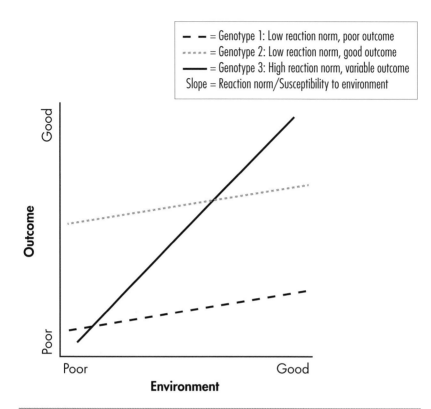

FIGURE 2–1. **Representation of changes in loneliness in different genotypes across varying environmental conditions.**

Genotypes 1 and 2 show relatively stable loneliness responses. Genotype 3 shows greater loneliness reactivity across varying environmental conditions. This model illustrates that a high reactivity genotype may be more beneficial than other genotypes under highly favorable conditions but may be more detrimental under adverse conditions.

Source. Adapted with permission of Sage Publications, from "Genetic Contributions to Loneliness and Their Relevance to the Evolutionary Theory of Loneliness." *Perspectives on Psychological Science*, Vol 14(3), pp 376–396, 2019. Permission conveyed through Copyright Clearance Center, Inc.

Social Connection and Loneliness

Research in loneliness has often been tied to its corresponding effects on human health and well-being. Therefore, it is important to contextualize loneliness among other social factors represented in the broader health literature. *Social connection* is an umbrella term that encompasses the full scope of measurement approaches used in the broader literature, each of which aims to capture the ways in which social relationships, or lack thereof, may influence health and health relevant outcomes (Holt-Lunstad 2018; Holt-

Lunstad et al. 2017). Because this literature emerged across various scientific disciplines, multiple perspectives, terms, and measurement approaches similarly emerged. Across these approaches, some measurements are aimed at assessing social assets (e.g., social support), whereas others are focused on assessing social deficits (e.g., loneliness).

Table 2–2 provides definitions for several common terms in this literature, including definitions for the three key components of social connection shown to significantly impact human health: social isolation, loneliness, and social support. *Social isolation* is the *objective* lack or limited extent of social ties or contacts with others. These social ties are usually defined as the marriage/partnership relationship, relationships with friends and relatives, and membership in religious or community groups. *Loneliness* is the *subjective* feeling or perception of being socially isolated. This occurs when the quantity or quality of one's social relationships is experienced as deficient. *Perceived loneliness* and *loneliness* are equivalent terms. Although social isolation has been shown to increase risk for loneliness, they do not always co-occur. Objective and subjective measures of isolation are only weakly correlated in population-based studies ($r=0.2$) (Cornwell and Waite 2009; Donovan et al. 2017). *Social support* refers to the availability of social resources that can be either *subjectively* or *objectively* appraised. These include provisions of emotional support, tangible help (i.e., instrumental support), or information and advice (i.e., informational support).

Social Relationship Assets and Deficits

With a few exceptions, most social connection measures are scored and analyzed on a continuum. Thus, depending on how the questions are framed, a particular measurement approach could represent a continuum of assets and deficits. For example, high scores on the Berkman-Syme Social Network Index (Berkman and Syme 1979) have been used to examine the protective effects of social integration, whereas low scores have been used to identify risk associated with social isolation (see chapter appendix). *Social engagement* is another term related to social network and social integration that has an opposite polarity with social isolation (see Table 2–2). Most measurement approaches to loneliness can be viewed as a subjective assessment of social deficits rather than a continuum of assets and deficits.

Structure, Function, and Quality Aspects of Social Relationships

Varied approaches in the health literature can be generally categorized as measuring assets or deficits across the structure, function, and quality of so-

TABLE 2–2.   **Social connection and related terms**

Social connection	Umbrella term encompassing the structural, functional, and quality aspects of human relationships
Social isolation	Objective lack or limited extent of social ties or contacts with others; broad structural category of social connection
Social integration	Extent of social ties or contacts with others; reciprocal term to *social isolation*
Social networks	Extent or density of social ties based on marital, family/relative, and group ties
Social engagement	Frequency of contacts with family/relatives, friends, and religious or community groups
Loneliness	Subjective feeling or perception of being socially isolated; quantity and quality of social relationships experienced as deficient; corresponds most closely to functional and quality aspects of social connections
Social support	Actual or perceived availability of resources from relationships (emotional, instrumental/tangible, or informational forms of support); broad functional category of social connection
Received support	Self-reported receipt of support
Perceived support	Perception of available support if needed
Other terms	
Social exclusion	Experience of being disregarded or rejected by others
Belonging or belongingness	Subjective experience of having relationships that bring about a secure sense of fitting in
Relationship strain	Subjective ratings of conflict, distress, or ambivalence

cial relationships (Figure 2–2). Evidence suggests that each of these aspects of social relationships may independently contribute to health and well-being.

Structure

Many of the earliest and most established measurement approaches examine the structure of how we connect to others socially. These types of measures tend to be more objective and quantifiable. For example, measures of the structure of one's social connections may assess the size or diversity of one's social network or one's social roles, frequency of social contact, number of people in one's household, or number or frequency of participation

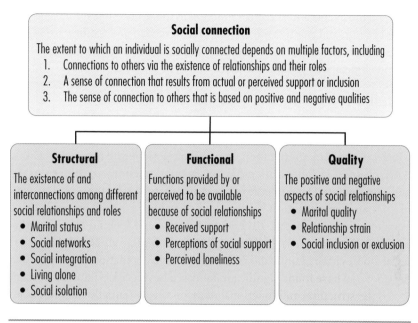

FIGURE 2–2.   Structural, functional, and quality components of social connection.

Source.   Reproduced with permission from Holt-Lunstad J: "Why Social Relationships Are Important for Physical Health: A Systems Approach to Understanding and Modifying Risk and Protection." *Annual Review of Psychology* 69:437–458, 2018 29035688. Permission conveyed through Copyright Clearance Center, Inc.

in social groups. *Social isolation*, *social integration*, and *social engagement* are terms that fall within this domain of social connection. The existence of, proximity to, and regular contact with others provides the structural foundation on which the functions and quality of these relationships may operate. Thus, absence or insufficiency in this domain may limit the opportunity to reap benefits in other domains (Holt-Lunstad and Steptoe 2021).

Function

Some measurement approaches examine our connections to others via the functions that those relationships serve. The functional component of social connection captures this connection to others through the actual resources they provide us or the resources we perceive to be available to meet our various needs, such as emotional, physical, tangible, informational, and belonging needs. These types of measures can be relatively objective or subjective. For example, social support measurement can include both the objectively received social support and the subjective perceptions of received or available social support. Social support provides resources and buffering during stressful life events and enhances function in the context of exploration, goal achievement, and positive life events (Pietromonaco and Collins 2017). So-cial support has been widely examined in relation to health outcomes both within clinical settings and without.

Quality

Despite the many benefits associated with social relationships, not all rela-tionships are positive. Thus, it is also important to distinguish the extent to which our connections to others vary in their positive and negative qualities. Such measures include relationship satisfaction, cohesion, adjustment, strain, and ambivalence. Data have shown that negativity in relationships (e.g., con-flict, strain, neglect, abuse) has been linked to poorer health and well-being outcomes (Friedman et al. 2012; Holt-Lunstad and Uchino 2019; Lund et al. 2014; Pietromonaco and Powers 2015; Robles et al. 2014). Relatively fewer studies have examined this domain in large populations, but those that have done so have found significant increased health risks. Thus, assessment across the structural and functional domains can potentially miss risk asso-ciated with poor-quality relationships. Furthermore, well-intentioned in-terventions that increase social contact as a means of reducing loneliness without attending to the *quality* of that social contact may result in unin-tended harm.

When examining objective health outcomes, including mortality, mor-bidity, and biomarkers, evidence supports the predictive utility of each of these measurement approaches. The correlations between these measures are not high, suggesting that each component may be important in predict-ing risk and may tap into unique pathways. Data from four nationally rep-resentative samples across the life span suggest that structure, function, and quality predict biomarkers and longevity in a dose-response manner (Yang et al. 2016). These data also indicate that the importance of each domain differs vastly according to stage of life. For example, relationship quality was a much stronger predictor of inflammation in adolescents, whereas structure of relationships was a stronger predictor of inflammatory markers among older adults.

Where Does Loneliness Fit Within the Structure, Function, and Quality Framework?

Although loneliness is clearly an indicator of social deficits, does it align conceptually within one or more of these aspects of social connection? Nearly every definition of loneliness describes it as subjective, thus, it is relatively clear that loneliness is not an objective indicator of social deficits (e.g., social isolation) nor does it fall under the broad categorization of a "structural" component of social connection. However, given its subjectivity, loneliness *could* conceptually represent perceived inadequacies in relationships meeting needs (functions) or perceived dissatisfaction with relationships (quality). In some examples of social connection frameworks, loneliness has been identified as falling under the functional domain of social connection (see Figure 2–2) (Holt-Lunstad 2018). However, it may have relevance for and applicability to the quality domain.

In Perlman and Peplau's (1981) original description, loneliness was characterized as "the unpleasant experience that occurs when a person's network of social relations is deficient in some important way, either quantitatively or qualitatively" (p. 31). Thus, loneliness may represent problems in the emotional satisfaction obtained from relationships or the functional benefits of social relationships, encompassing the spectrum of emotional, social, and collective forms of loneliness. It follows that loneliness should prompt an evaluation of past and current relationship quality and a possible history of deprivation or other emotionally harmful relationship experiences. To remediate certain conditions of loneliness, there may be opportunities to repair or enhance the quality of existing relationships by attending to capacities for intimacy, affection, and love (Pietromonaco and Collins 2017).

Representative Measures of Social Connection

Because of the manifold associations of social isolation and loneliness with poorer mental and physical health, expert consensus recommends screening for both in health care settings and including measures for these social conditions in all electronic health records (Institute of Medicine 2014; National Academies of Sciences, Engineering, and Medicine 2020). For example, the National Academies of Sciences, Engineering, and Medicine (NASEM) report in 2020 recommended screening older adults for social isolation and loneliness in all primary and specialty health care practices and settings. This report acknowledged important limitations of and questions about proper implementation of currently available measurement scales. Nearly all measurement scales have been designed for use in research studies, and most measures lack defined cut points for routine clinical screening. Furthermore, the evidence base for interventions for these conditions is limited, which complicates practitioners' ability to respond properly.

Despite these limitations, there are certain practical approaches to the assessment of social isolation and loneliness. A practical first step is to screen for and monitor social isolation and loneliness using one of the available validated measurement scales and to routinely ask about these social concerns in the clinical encounter. Despite the absence of a clear cut point for loneliness, responses during screening can be a starting point for further inquiry, and longitudinal scores can be informative. Practical approaches also include recognizing high-risk factors, such as developmental or phase-of-life changes, relationship loss, a geographical move, or health conditions that impair social connection, such as hearing loss, mental health disorders, or stigmatizing medical conditions (see Table 2–1). This level of under-standing may point to logical interventions or further steps to ameliorate social isolation or loneliness. Approaches specific to patients with mental health conditions and to younger and older people are presented in Chapter 4 ("Loneliness in People Living With Mental Health Disorders"), Chapter 8 ("Interventions for Loneliness in Younger People"), and Chapter 9 ("Interventions for Loneliness in Older Adults").

Mental health practitioners are well-equipped to recognize individual differences involved in the genesis and persistence of loneliness. These important differences may spring from personality factors, such as neuroticism or introversion, or from formative life experiences, current life circumstances, or relationship experiences with family, peers, and romantic partners. During this process of inquiry, it is important to clarify actual relationship deficits, to recognize the nature of any perceived relationship deficits (e.g., emotional, social, or collective loneliness), and to note attributions to loneliness and cognitive biases. Susceptibility to loneliness and its subtypes would be expected to vary based on these individual differences and across life stages.

To aid in the identification and monitoring of loneliness and other aspects of social connection, several measurement scales are presented in the appendix to this chapter. The Center for Epidemiologic Studies Depression scale (Radloff 1977) contains a single question about loneliness that has been used as a direct self-reported measure of loneliness. Generally, this measurement approach is not preferred because its direct use of the word *lonely* may elicit a stigmatizing reaction and biased response, leading to underreporting (Boyrs 1985).

Commonly used loneliness scales are versions of the UCLA LS and the De Jong Gierveld Loneliness Scale. The UCLA LS, Version 3 (UCLA LS3) is composed of 20 items (Russell 1996) and is considered the gold standard version of this scale. A 4-item version composed of items 1, 13, 15, and 18 from the larger version has also been validated as a shortened scale (Russell et al. 1980). Readers can view the questions and response format for these scales by referring to Russell (1996) and Russell et al. (1980). A 3-item version of the UCLA LS (Hughes et al. 2004) is included in the chapter appendix; it has been widely implemented in large population-based studies and was recommended in the NASEM report for implementation in electronic health records (National Academies of Sciences, Engineering, and Medicine 2020). The 4-item version of the UCLA LS is considered to have more favorable psychometric properties than the 3-item version based on its inclusion of both positively and negatively worded items and its four-point rather than three-point response format. The 6-item De Jong Gierveld scale is often used because of its validated subscales for emotional and social loneliness, as noted in the chapter appendix. Other scales for loneliness are freely available to the public via the National Institutes of Health (NIH)'s Health Measures website (www.healthmeasures.net). For example, the Patient-Reported Outcomes Measurement Information System (PROMIS) 8-item loneliness scale, entitled "Social Isolation," is increasingly used in research studies (see chapter appendix).

The NASEM report cautioned against the use of scales that are not validated (National Academies of Sciences, Engineering, and Medicine 2020). In addition, NASEM emphasized choosing a measurement scale designed for the specific aspect of social connection under study, because measures for loneliness, social isolation, social support, and other social constructs are not interchangeable.

Representative measures for social isolation and social support are presented in the chapter appendix to exemplify these other aspects of social connection. The Berkman-Syme Social Network Index is a framework for measuring social integration or social isolation that has been adapted and implemented in many forms. The Steptoe Social Isolation Index (Steptoe et al. 2013) builds on this framework and provides a quantitative cut point for social isolation. These scales are most applicable to adult samples. Examples of NIH health measures specific for emotional, informational, and instrumental support are also shown. Other well-known measures of global social support include the Interpersonal Support Evaluation List (Cohen and Hoberman 1983) and abbreviated versions of the Duke Social Support Scale (Koenig et al. 1993), although the latter incorporate a combination of structural, functional, and quality items.

Case Vignette

Virginia is a 75-year-old woman with history of recurrent major depression who experienced an episode of severe depression during the SARS-CoV-2 (COVID-19) pandemic, shortly after her husband died from long-term complications of a stroke.

Virginia never knew her father, who had died in a motor vehicle accident 6 months before she was born. Her mother was unaffectionate, strict, and controlling. Virginia was raised with three siblings and half-siblings. She experienced a first episode of depression during high school but did not receive treatment. During college, she took an academic leave for outpatient and later residential treatment of depression that consisted of psychotherapy. As a young woman, she was married and raised four children in a close-knit family. Episodes of recurrent depression were treated with serotonin reuptake inhibitors and psychotherapy. Although she describes herself as an introvert, she has had longstanding friendships and was an active community volunteer, visiting homebound elderly persons and those struggling with chronic illnesses. She also participated in a community chorus.

In the year prior to COVID-19, Virginia moved from the home where she had raised her family to live in an apartment near her son and his family in the same suburban town. At that time, her depression was treated with a combination of a serotonin reuptake inhibitor and mirtazapine, and she was euthymic. During the early pandemic, she thought that she was managing well. Her husband was in skilled nursing care, where she visited him regularly until his death 9 months into the pandemic. During visits with her husband, she would often sing songs that they had enjoyed during their lives. One month after his death, she began to experience what she described as characteristic depressive symptoms: low energy, low motivation, excessive sleep, and tearfulness.

Over the ensuing months, Virginia's depression worsened, with persistently depressed mood, prominent anhedonia, frequent crying, difficulty concentrating, poor appetite, feelings of dread, and avoidance of social activities. Her depression (Patient Health Questionnaire–9) and loneliness (PROMIS Isolation 8a) scores were consistent with severe depression and moderate loneliness. Pharmacological changes included a switch to a serotonin-norepinephrine reuptake inhibitor in combination with mirtazapine and adjunctive gabapentin. Psychiatric treatment also included psychoeducation about grief symptoms following spousal loss, its natural history, and adaptive processes involved in the resolution of grief.

Virginia engaged in telehealth-delivered cognitive-behavioral therapy with a focus on behavioral activation approach and theory. This treatment promoted value-based action despite lower motivation and giving credit to this action no matter the outcome. It evoked value-based language behind her actions, including thoughtfulness and helping others, gratitude, having moments of respite and the freedom of her imagination, courageousness, and engaging in music in a way that connects people. Socialization was an important treatment focus because she dreaded social events when she was depressed, compounding the social disruption of her move and the social restrictions of the pandemic. By increasing her effort to socially engage, Virginia became more aware of her desire for connection and the benefit of follow-up interactions that naturally occur.

During this period, she also participated in a research study of music therapy for older adults experiencing loneliness during COVID-19. During eight weekly sessions with a certified music therapist, she developed relaxing and energizing personal music playlists using an online subscription. Virginia experienced a close personal connection to the music therapist, who encouraged her to listen to both of her playlists daily and to reflect on her experience of the music, how it affected her mood and breathing, the memories it elicited, and the songs that resonated with her during the week. She was particularly captivated by music from participants in televised singing competitions. Songs such as "You Raise Me Up" and "You'll Never Walk Alone" brought her comfort or elicited memories of her late husband and her father. She was inspired by the life stories of the contestants on these programs and by their music: "It opens me up and brings something out of me that may be closed off.... I put myself in the shoes of whoever is singing the words. It takes me away from whatever is in my head to another place. It's fun to hear the voices."

This vignette describes a picture of relationship loss and emotional loneliness in early childhood and the development of severe depression beginning in late adolescence. It also presents a story of resilience, a woman who built stable emotional, social, and community connections through her marriage, family, neighbors, and friends; a love of music; empathy for others; and meaningful community volunteerism. When Virginia experienced acute social disconnection and severe depression due to COVID-19 and the loss of her husband, her recovery was scaffolded by the emotional, informational, practical, and therapeutic support of her treatment team. Through music she felt supported because it made her think of her husband and her father. She identified with the courage of the musicians and was soothed by the beauty and meaning of their music.

Summary

This chapter reviews the theoretical basis of loneliness as a state of social and psychological distress based on basic human needs for intimate connection, sustaining social relations, and collective engagement with others. Loneliness is subjective in nature, a deficit in the desired quantity or quality of one's social relationships. Original descriptions of loneliness and its antecedent factors remain accurate and relevant today. Well-established measures of loneliness are available.

Genetic studies have provided critical insights into individual differences in susceptibility to loneliness under conditions of social stress. These differences within a population can be viewed as a form of behavioral diversity that is adaptive to societies under varying environmental conditions. Coheritability with traits such as neuroticism and, to a lesser extent, introversion have been most consistently noted in genetic studies. Thus, the experience of loneliness is a product of the genetic predisposition and accumulated experience of an individual interacting with current stresses and social resources.

It is useful to distinguish loneliness from other components of social connection, a term that broadly encompasses the structural, functional, and quality aspects of social relationships. Loneliness is conceptually distinct from social isolation (the objective lack or limited extent of social relationships) and social support (the provisions of social relationships). In life, however, loneliness is influenced by these other structural, functional, and quality components of relationships.

KEY POINTS

- Loneliness is the product of individual susceptibility to loneliness, arising from genetic, developmental, cognitive, and other person-specific factors interacting with exogenous social stresses. Some individuals are more reactive to positive and negative social stimuli than others.

- Varying susceptibilities to loneliness within a population represent a form of social behavioral diversity that is proposed to be adaptive for societies as a whole. Thus, individual responses to social stresses are not uniform and call for personalized approaches.

- Loneliness is a subjective but measurable psychometric construct with emotional, social, and collective components representing basic human needs for intimacy, friendship, and group affiliation.

- Concepts such as *social connection* (an overarching term related to social relationships), *loneliness*, *social isolation*, and *social support* are all well-established in the health literature. Other concepts and corresponding terms (e.g., *social rejection* or *exclusion*, *relationship strain*, *negativity/hostility*, *ambivalence*, *belonging*) allow for a more complete understanding of the social relationship structures, functions, and qualities that cumulatively and interactively impact human health.

Suggested Readings

Cacioppo JT, Cacioppo S: The phenotype of loneliness. Eur J Dev Psychol 9(4):446–452, 2012

Holt-Lunstad J: Why social relationships are important for physical health: a systems approach to understanding and modifying risk and protection. Annu Rev Psychol 69:437–458, 2018

National Academies of Sciences, Engineering, and Medicine: Social Isolation and Loneliness in Older Adults: Opportunities for the Health Care System. Washington, DC, The National Academies Press, 2020

Perissinotto C, Holt-Lunstad J, Periyakoil VS, Covinsky K: A practical approach to assessing and mitigating loneliness and isolation in older adults. J Am Geriatr Soc 67(4):657–662, 2019

References

Abdellaoui A, Nivard MG, Hottenga JJ, et al: Predicting loneliness with polygenic scores of social, psychological and psychiatric traits. Genes Brain Behav 17(6):e12472, 2018 29573219

Berkman LF, Syme SL: Social networks, host resistance, and mortality: a nine-year follow-up study of Alameda County residents. Am J Epidemiol 109(2):186–204, 1979 425958

Boyrs SPD: Gender differences in loneliness. Pers Soc Psychol Bull 11(1):63–74, 1985

Cacioppo JT, Cacioppo S: The phenotype of loneliness. Eur J Dev Psychol 9(4):446–452, 2012 23024688

Cacioppo JT, Cacioppo S, Boomsma DI: Evolutionary mechanisms for loneliness. Cogn Emotion 28(1):3–21, 2014 24067110

Cohen S, Hoberman H: Positive events and social supports as buffers of life change stress. J Appl Soc Psychol 13(2):99–125, 1983

Cornwell EY, Waite LJ: Measuring social isolation among older adults using multiple indicators from the NSHAP study. J Gerontol B Psychol Sci Soc Sci 64(suppl 1):i38–i46, 2009 19508982

De Jong Gierveld J: Developing and testing a model of loneliness. J Pers Soc Psychol 53(1):119–128, 1987 3612484

De Jong Gierveld J, Van Tilburg T: A 6-item scale for overall, emotional, and social loneliness. Research on Aging 28(5):582–598, 2006

Donovan NJ, Wu Q, Rentz DM, et al: Loneliness, depression and cognitive function in older U.S. adults. Int J Geriatr Psychiatry 32(5):564–573, 2017 27162047

Friedman EM, Karlamangla AS, Almeida DM, Seeman TE: Social strain and cortisol regulation in midlife in the US. Soc Sci Med 74(4):607–615, 2012 22209675

Fromm-Reichmann F: Loneliness. Psychiatry 22(1):1–15, 1959 13634274

Gao J, Davis LK, Hart AB, et al: Genome-wide association study of loneliness demonstrates a role for common variation. Neuropsychopharmacology 42(4):811–821, 2017

Hawkley LC, Browne MW, Cacioppo JT: How can I connect with thee? Let me count the ways. Psychol Sci 16(10):798–804, 2005 16181443

Holt-Lunstad J: Why social relationships are important for physical health: a systems approach to understanding and modifying risk and protection. Annu Rev Psychol 69:437–458, 2018 29035688

Holt-Lunstad J, Steptoe A: Social isolation: an underappreciated determinant of physical health. Curr Opin Psychol 43:232–237, 2021 34438331

Holt-Lunstad J, Uchino BN: Social ambivalence and disease (SAD): a theoretical model aimed at understanding the health implications of ambivalent relationships. Perspect Psychol Sci 14(6):941–966, 2019 31533019

Holt-Lunstad J, Robles TF, Sbarra DA: Advancing social connection as a public health priority in the United States. Am Psychol 72(6):517–530, 2017 28880099

Hughes ME, Waite LJ, Hawkley LC, Cacioppo JT: A short scale for measuring loneliness in large surveys: results from two population-based studies. Res Aging 26(6):655–672, 2004 18504506

Institute of Medicine: Capturing Social and Behavioral Domains and Measures in Electronic Health Records: Phase 2. Washington, DC, National Academies Press, 2014

Koenig HG, Westlund RE, George LK, et al: Abbreviating the Duke Social Support Index for use in chronically ill elderly individuals. Psychosomatics 34(1):61–69, 1993 8426892

Lund R, Christensen U, Nilsson CJ, et al: Stressful social relations and mortality: a prospective cohort study. J Epidemiol Community Health 68(8):720–727, 2014 24811775

Moustakas CE: Loneliness. Englewood Cliffs, NJ, Prentice-Hall, 1961

National Academies of Sciences, Engineering, and Medicine: Social Isolation and Loneliness in Older Adults: Opportunities for the Health Care System. Washington, DC, National Academies Press, 2020

Perlman DP, Peplau LA: Toward a social psychology of loneliness, in Personal Relationships, Vol 3: Relationships in Disorder. Edited by Duck SG, Gilmour R. London, Academic Press, 1981, pp 31–56

Pietromonaco PR, Collins NL: Interpersonal mechanisms linking close relationships to health. Am Psychol 72(6):531–542, 2017 28880100

Pietromonaco PR, Powers SI: Attachment and health-related physiological stress processes. Curr Opin Psychol 1:34–39, 2015 25729755

Qualter P, Vanhalst J, Harris R, et al: Loneliness across the life span. Perspect Psychol Sci 10(2):250–264, 2015 25910393

Radloff LS: The CES-D Scale: a self-report depression scale for research in the general population. Appl Psychol Meas 1(3):385–401, 1977

Robles TF, Slatcher RB, Trombello JM, McGinn MM: Marital quality and health: a meta-analytic review. Psychol Bull 140(1):140–187, 2014 23527470

Russell DW: UCLA Loneliness Scale (Version 3): reliability, validity, and factor structure. J Pers Assess 66(1):20–40, 1996 8576833

Russell DW, Peplau LA, Ferguson ML: Developing a measure of loneliness. J Pers Assess 42(3):290–294, 1978 660402

Russell DW, Peplau LA, Cutrona CE: The revised UCLA Loneliness Scale: concurrent and discriminant validity evidence. J Pers Soc Psychol 39(3):472–480, 1980 7431205

Spithoven AWM, Cacioppo S, Goossens L, Cacioppo JT: Genetic contributions to loneliness and their relevance to the evolutionary theory of loneliness. Perspect Psychol Sci 14(3):376–396, 2019 30844327

Steptoe A, Shankar A, Demakakos P, Wardle J: Social isolation, loneliness, and all-cause mortality in older men and women. Proc Natl Acad Sci USA 110(15):5797–5801, 2013 23530191

Weiss RS: Loneliness: The Experience of Emotional and Social Isolation. Cambridge, MA, MIT Press, 1973

Yang YC, Boen C, Gerken K, et al: Social relationships and physiological determinants of longevity across the human life span. Proc Natl Acad Sci USA 113(3):578–583, 2016 26729882

Appendix of Measures

The following are representative instruments that have been validated or empirically used for measuring loneliness, social isolation, and social support. These scales were reformatted for use in this appendix.

Loneliness Measures

1. Center for Epidemiological Studies–Depression Scale (CES-D) single-item loneliness measure
2. Three-item UCLA Loneliness Scale (20-item and 4-item versions of this scale can be found in Russell 1996 and Russell et al. 1980).
3. Six-item De Jong Gierveld Scale for Loneliness
4. Patient-Reported Outcomes Measurement Information System (PROMIS)—Isolation Short-Form 8a

Social Isolation Measures

1. Steptoe Social Isolation Index
2. Berkman-Syme Social Network Index

Social Support Measures

1. PROMIS Emotional Support—Short Form 4a
2. PROMIS Informational Support—Short Form 4a
3. PROMIS Instrumental Support—Short Form 4a

For additional publicly available NIH-sponsored measures, visit www.healthmeasures.net/explore-measurement-systems/promis and then select "Search and View" measures under the domain "Relationships/Social Support." Pediatric measures are available at this site, as are translated instruments.

Loneliness Measures

Center for Epidemiological Studies–Depression Scale (CES-D) Single-Item Loneliness Measure

During the past week:

I felt lonely:	Rarely or none of the time	Some or a little of the time	Occasionally or a moderate amount of time	Most or all of the time
	<1 day	1–2 days	3–4 days	5–7 days

Note. This single question is derived from the CES-D scale and has been used to measure loneliness in some epidemiological studies that lack a validated loneliness scale.

Source. Radloff 1977; publicly available scale.

Three-item UCLA Loneliness Scale

1. How often do you feel you lack companionship?	Hardly ever (1)	Some of the time (2)	Often (3)
2. How often do you feel left out?	Hardly ever (1)	Some of the time (2)	Often (3)
3. How often do you feel isolated from others?	Hardly ever (1)	Some of the time (2)	Often (3)

Note. A continuous measure of loneliness. Total score is calculated as the sum of the three item scores; higher score indicates greater loneliness.

Source. Adapted with permission of Sage Publications, from "A Short Scale for Measuring Loneliness in Large Surveys: Results From Two Population-Based Studies." *Research on Aging*, Vol 26(6), pp. 655–672, 2004. Permission conveyed through Copyright Clearance Center, Inc.

Six-Item De Jong Gierveld Scale for Loneliness

	Yes	More or Less	No
1. I feel a general sense of emptiness.	❑	❑	❑
2. I miss having people around.	❑	❑	❑
3. I often feel rejected.	❑	❑	❑
4. There are plenty of people I can rely on when I have problems.	❑	❑	❑
5. There are many people I can trust completely.	❑	❑	❑
6. There are enough people I feel close to.	❑	❑	❑

Items 1–3, Emotional Loneliness subscale. Scoring Yes=3, More or less=2, No=1.
Items 4–6, Social Loneliness subscale. Scoring Yes=1, More or less=2, No=3.
Total score=sum of subscale scores (possible range, 6–18). Higher score indicates greater loneliness for subscale scores and total score.

Source. Adapted with permission of Sage Publications, from "A 6-Item Scale for Overall, Emotional, and Social Loneliness." *Research on Aging*, Vol 28(5), pp. 582–598, 2006. Permission conveyed through Copyright Clearance Center, Inc.

PROMIS Isolation—Short Form 8a

	Never	Rarely	Sometimes	Usually	Always
1. I feel left out:	1	2	3	4	5
2. I feel that people barely know me:	1	2	3	4	5
3. I feel isolated from others:	1	2	3	4	5
4. I feel that people are around me but not with me:	1	2	3	4	5
5. I feel isolated even when I am not alone:	1	2	3	4	5
6. I feel that people avoid talking to me:	1	2	3	4	5
7. I feel detached from other people:	1	2	3	4	5
8. I feel like a stranger to those around me:	1	2	3	4	5

Note. Higher score indicates greater loneliness. For further scoring instructions, visit www.promishealth.org/healthmeasures. This measure is publicly available without license.

Social Isolation Measures

Steptoe Social Isolation Index

Five-item scale, with one point being assigned for each of the following items:

1. Being unmarried or not cohabitating
2. Less than monthly contact with children (face-to-face, by telephone or writing/email)
3. Less than monthly contact with other family (face-to-face, by telephone or writing/email)
4. Less than monthly contact with friends (face-to-face, by telephone or writing/email)
5. No participation in social clubs, resident groups, religious groups, or committees

Note.   A score of 2 or more is defined as socially isolated.

Source.   Steptoe et al. 2013.

Berkman-Syme Social Network Index

A measure of social ties and contacts based on domains of marriage/partnership, contacts with family and friends, participation in religious organizations, and community groups. Has been widely adapted and implemented in epidemiological surveys.

Illustrative questions

1. In a typical week how often do you talk on the telephone with family, friends, or neighbors?
2. How often do you get together with friends and relatives?
3. How often do you attend church or religious services?
4. How often do you attend meetings of clubs or organizations that you belong to?

Marital status is assessed separately and used in scoring.

Note.   Higher score indicates higher social integration and less social isolation. Many variations of this measure have been used.

Source.   Berkman and Syme 1979; National Academies of Sciences, Engineering, and Medicine 2020.

Social Support Measures

PROMIS Emotional Support—Short Form 4a

	Never	Rarely	Sometimes	Usually	Always
1. I have someone who will listen to me when I need to talk:	1	2	3	4	5
2. I have someone to confide in or talk to about myself or my problems:	1	2	3	4	5
3. I have someone who makes me feel appreciated:	1	2	3	4	5
4. I have someone to talk with when I have a bad day:	1	2	3	4	5

Note. Higher score indicates greater emotional support. For further scoring instructions, visit www.promishealth.org/healthmeasures. This measure is publicly available without license.

PROMIS Informational Support—Short Form 4a

	Never	Rarely	Sometimes	Usually	Always
1. I have someone to give me good advice about a crisis if I need it:	1	2	3	4	5
2. I have someone to turn to for suggestions about how to deal with a problem:	1	2	3	4	5
3. I have someone to give me information if I need it:	1	2	3	4	5
4. I get useful advice about important things in life:	1	2	3	4	5

Note. Higher score indicates greater informational support. For further scoring instructions, visit www.promishealth.org/healthmeasures. This measure is publicly available without license.

PROMIS Instrumental Support—Short Form 4a

	Never	Rarely	Sometimes	Usually	Always
1. Do you have someone to help you if you are confined to bed?	1	2	3	4	5
2. Do you have someone to take you to the doctor if you need it?	1	2	3	4	5
3. Do you have someone to help you with your daily chores if you are sick?	1	2	3	4	5
4. Do you have someone to run errands if you need it?	1	2	3	4	5

Note.   Higher score indicates greater instrumental support. For further scoring instructions, visit www.promishealth.org/healthmeasures. This measure is publicly available without license.

3

Loneliness Across the Life Span

Maike Luhmann, Ph.D.
Louise Hawkley, Ph.D.
Susanne Buecker, Ph.D.
Tilmann von Soest, Ph.D.
Jürgen Margraf, Ph.D.

PEOPLE FEEL LONELY when the quality and quantity of their social relationships and social interactions do not meet what they desire (Peplau and Perlman 1982). Given this definition, it is perhaps not surprising that many people associate loneliness primarily with a time in life at which social relationships tend to be objectively scarce: old age. Old age is characterized by the loss of a spouse, friends, or functional health. These kinds of losses impair older adults' opportunities for social interactions and may lead to loneliness.

However, loneliness is by no means restricted to later life but can occur at any age and for reasons not limited to objective losses of social contact and

The authors would like to thank Marilena Rüsberg for her assistance in the literature search.

interactions. Rather, predictors of loneliness vary across the life span. This observation has important implications for individual- and community-level interventions targeted at preventing and combating loneliness and may have implications for health consequences associated with loneliness.

In this chapter we discuss loneliness from a life-span perspective. We begin with a brief overview of definitions and measurements of loneliness and discuss conceptual and methodological issues that must be considered when studying loneliness across the life span. We then review empirical findings on the distribution of loneliness and its predictors and health outcomes. We end with a discussion of the implications for prevention and intervention.

Definition and Measurement of Loneliness

Loneliness is commonly defined as a perceived discrepancy between individuals' desired and actual social relationships (Peplau and Perlman 1982; see Chapter 2, "Loneliness, Other Aspects of Social Connection, and Their Measurement"). The term *perceived* highlights that loneliness is a subjective experience. In contrast, *social isolation* is the objective state of having no or few social connections. Social isolation and loneliness are related but distinct: people can feel lonely despite having a large social network, and socially isolated people can be completely content and not lonely despite their isolation. As a general tendency, however, socially isolated people are more likely to feel lonely than non-isolated people.

Loneliness is usually measured using self-report questionnaires (see Chapter 2). Most large-scale panel studies use direct measures consisting of a single item, such as "During the past 4 weeks, how often have you felt lonely?" and offering response options such as "Never," "Rarely," "Often," and "Most or all of the time." These measures typically assess the frequency of loneliness and are direct because the term *lonely* is used. Direct single-item measures are face-valid and economical but have been criticized because the word *lonely* can be stigmatized and might lead to biased responses (Borys and Perlman 1985). Gender differences have been reported in responses to direct versus indirect measures of loneliness and for specific age groups (Maes et al. 2019).

Many empirical studies therefore rely on multi-item indirect measures that avoid *lonely* (De Jong Gierveld and van Tilburg 2006; Russell 1996). These measures assess the frequency or intensity of loneliness and sometimes measure more than one facet of loneliness. For example, the six-item De Jong Gierveld Scale (De Jong Gierveld and van Tilburg 2006) can be used to generate two separate scores, one for emotional loneliness and another for social loneliness. *Emotional loneliness* refers to the perceived lack of a close confidant or significant other. *Social loneliness* refers to the perceived lack of close relationships with friends, family, or neighbors. Indirect multi-item measures allow a more fine-grained and reliable assessment of loneliness than single-item measures, but lay people may find them to be less intuitive in their interpretation. Studies comparing these measures across age groups generally find them to be reliable and valid (Danneel et al. 2018; Maes et al. 2015), which is crucial for studies of loneliness across the life span because it suggests that mean-level comparisons using these measures across age groups are permissible and meaningful.

Regardless of whether loneliness is measured in terms of frequency or intensity, it is usually considered a continuous variable. In some fields (e.g., medicine) and for some research objectives (e.g., to assess the prevalence of loneliness in a population or across the life course), a simple binary distinction between "lonely" and "non-lonely" people is sometimes preferred. To achieve such a distinction, the continuous loneliness distribution must be dichotomized—that is, a specific score on the continuum must be chosen as a cutoff that divides the sample into these two groups. There is no standardized approach to choosing this cutoff; some studies use a conservative cutoff that only counts as "lonely" those who feel lonely most of the time (e.g., Yang and Victor 2011), whereas other studies use a more lenient cutoff that also includes people who feel lonely sometimes (in terms of frequency) or moderately (in terms of intensity) (e.g., Franssen et al. 2020). The more lenient approach thus results in higher loneliness prevalence estimates than the conservative approach. Overall, binary measures of loneliness are appealing because they provide prevalence estimates of loneliness that are easier to interpret than some arbitrary scale score. However, the lack of a standardized cutoff complicates comparisons of results across studies. The arbitrary dichotomization also leads to a loss in variance, which means that subtle changes in the loneliness distribution (e.g., people moving from "never lonely" to "sometimes lonely") remain undetected. These caveats must be kept in mind when reviewing studies on age differences in loneliness.

Conceptual and Theoretical Perspectives

Some people are more likely to feel lonely than others, regardless of their specific circumstances. Twin studies indicate that loneliness is partly heritable, suggesting it has a genetic basis (Goossens et al. 2015). Loneliness is correlated with relatively stable personality traits such as neuroticism and extraversion (Buecker et al. 2020b) and is associated with attachment experiences in early childhood (Merz and Jak 2013). Longitudinal studies show that it is characterized by a relatively high rank-order stability (Böger and Huxhold 2018b) and that a substantial proportion of its stability over time can be explained by stable trait effects (Mund et al. 2020b). Together, these findings indicate that individual differences in loneliness are often dispositional. This does not mean that one's loneliness levels are carved in stone but simply that these levels are not completely determined by one's social environment. Loneliness can and does change across the life span.

Different Ways of Change

Change can be conceptualized in different ways (Mund et al. 2020a). *Rank-order change* refers to changes in a person's relative standing in comparison with others. This is typically measured by examining the correlation between loneliness scores measured at Time 1 and those measured at Time 2. A high correlation indicates high rank-order stability, which means that individuals who had higher-than-average loneliness levels at Time 1 are likely to also have higher-than-average loneliness levels at Time 2. Importantly, rank-order change only refers to whether individuals changed their position in the rank order, independent of whether their individual loneliness score changed. High rank-order stability is usually interpreted as a sign that a construct is trait-like, meaning that it is substantially influenced by stable characteristics of the person and less by more transient characteristics of the social environment (Mund et al. 2020b).

Mean-level change refers to changes in average loneliness levels in a population over time. For continuous variables, sample means are tracked across repeated occasions. For dichotomized variables, the proportion of people who are categorized as lonely is tracked across repeated occasions. In addition, it is possible to examine individual trajectories of loneliness over time and to examine to what extent these trajectories differ between individuals, for example, by identifying latent classes of people with distinct trajectories (Qualter et al. 2015; Schinka et al. 2013). In this chapter, we are particularly interested in how average levels of loneliness change across the life span and therefore primarily focus on studies of mean-level change.

Theoretical Explanations for Age Differences in Loneliness

Feeling connected to others is a fundamental human need (Baumeister and Leary 1995). *Fundamental* implies that this need exists from birth to death. People who do not feel connected to others may experience loneliness regardless of their age. Children as young as 6 years can have a basic understanding of what loneliness is (Asher and Paquette 2003). However, what it takes to feel connected does vary by age and is not uniformly distributed across age groups.

Loneliness levels might change over the life span because of changes in both the prevalence and the relevance of risk factors of loneliness (Luhmann and Hawkley 2016; von Soest et al. 2020b). *Prevalence* refers to the frequency with which a specific risk factor exists in a specific age group. For example, younger adults tend to have larger social networks than older adults (Sander et al. 2017), decreasing their risk for loneliness. The relative impact of a risk factor has been posited to be related to its *relevance* in a specific age group. For example, having a large social network is more important for adolescents and young adults than for older adults, so having a small social network may have a stronger effect on loneliness among younger than among older adults (Qualter et al. 2015).

As this example shows, the prevalence and relevance explanations are not mutually exclusive when applied to specific risk factors. For some risk factors, such as having a small social network, prevalence and relevance may develop in opposite directions across the life span (e.g., a risk factor becomes more common but at the same time less important with increasing age) and cancel each other out. For other risk factors, however, prevalence and relevance may develop in unison (e.g., a risk factor becomes more common and more important with increasing age). These risk factors may then contribute to loneliness more in certain age groups but less in others.

Relevance and prevalence can also influence each other. As some factors become less relevant with increasing age, people may invest less time and energy into sustaining them. For example, with increasing age, the importance of the *quantity* of friendships decreases, whereas the importance of the *quality* of friendships increases (Carmichael et al. 2015). People may therefore focus more on the quality of a few selected friendships and invest less time in sustaining a large network of acquaintances, thereby directly contributing to the changing prevalence of these factors over the life span (Sander et al. 2017).

Several psychological theories predict changes in the prevalence and relevance of risk factors across the life span. *Developmental theories* propose that different life stages are associated with different developmental tasks (Heckhausen et al. 2010; Qualter et al. 2015). Many developmental tasks are either directly aimed at establishing or maintaining specific social relationships or affect one's social relationships in indirect ways. In early childhood, the attachment to one's parents and immediate family is most important. In adolescence, relationships with one's peers and first romantic experiences become more central. Important developmental tasks in early adulthood include finding a partner, starting a family, and establishing a career. Middle adulthood is focused on maintaining and growing these social roles. Finally, old age is characterized not only by the loss of social partners but also by an increased focus on generativity (Heckhausen et al. 2010; Qualter et al. 2015). Hence, developmental theories allow some predictions about how the relevance of specific social relationships and other risk factors for loneliness change with time.

One developmental theory that is particularly relevant to understanding social relationships and loneliness across the life span is *socioemotional selectivity theory* (Carstensen et al. 1999). This theory proposes that older adults are more likely to perceive their remaining time as limited and hence focus more on emotional goals than do younger adults. Older adults are more likely to prioritize social relationships that they perceive as emotionally rewarding and to deprioritize those that are not rewarding. As a result, their social networks shrink in size but not in quality (Carstensen et al. 1999; Sander et al. 2017; Wrzus et al. 2013). Hence, socioemotional selectivity theory predicts that the prevalence of small social networks increases, but their relevance as predictors of loneliness decreases.

Finally, *biological changes* associated with aging must be considered when examining the prevalence of risk factors across the life span (Hawkley and Cacioppo 2007). Old age is characterized by decreasing health, increasing physical and sometimes cognitive limitations, and increasing frequency of deaths of partners and friends in one's age group. The elevated prevalence of these risk factors can contribute to elevated loneliness levels among the oldest old (Luhmann and Hawkley 2016).

Methodological Challenges in Studying the Life Span

Life span development can be studied with cross-sectional and longitudinal studies. Both approaches have strengths and limitations. *Cross-sectional studies* provide a snapshot of the loneliness distribution in a specific sample at a particular point in time. To provide meaningful age group comparisons, such studies must be based on samples that 1) represent different age groups with sufficient sample sizes and 2) are as representative as possible of the population of interest in terms of demographic characteristics such as sex, race/ethnicity, or socioeconomic status. In this chapter, we only discuss cross-sectional studies that meet these criteria.

Cross-sectional studies can be useful to identify age groups at particular risk for loneliness at the time of data collection and to examine predictors of loneliness across the life span. However, cross-sectional studies do not allow any conclusions about whether the observed age differences are due to age effects or cohort effects. For example, in one of our own studies using cross-sectional data from a large, nationally representative sample from Germany (Luhmann and Hawkley 2016), we found elevated loneliness levels among adults ages 30–35 years (discussed later). These elevated levels could be due to age effects, cohort effects, or both. It is possible that individuals between 30 and 35 years old are particularly prone to loneliness because this is a time in their life during which they must fulfill many demands (e.g., starting a family) that restrict their opportunities to maintain social activities (e.g., going out with their friends). This age-effect explanation implies that this age distribution should be replicable across different studies, regardless of whether the data were collected in 2013 (as was the case for this study) or in any other year. An alternative explanation for the elevated loneliness levels in this age group is that this particular generation (here, those born between 1978 and 1983) is more prone to loneliness than other generations, for example, because they were all subject to specific experiences that put them at a greater risk for loneliness at any age. This cohort-effect explanation implies that this specific population should have higher loneliness levels than those born a few years earlier or later, regardless of when their loneliness is measured.

Longitudinal studies follow individuals over time and measure their loneliness repeatedly. The number of measurement occasions and total study length can vary substantially, ranging from two occasions within a few months to multiple occasions spanning several decades. To study loneliness across the life span, longitudinal studies that measure loneliness multiple times over several years are more informative than those that cover only a few weeks or months. Longitudinal studies provide unique information about the development of loneliness across the life span that cannot be provided by cross-sectional studies. However, these studies are more challenging and expensive than cross-sectional studies, particularly if large representative samples are followed for longer periods of time. Longitudinal studies do not confound age and cohort effects, but they may confound age and period effects. *Period effects* refers to the effect of living during a specific period in history. For example, a longitudinal study that tracked young adults from 2019 to 2021 may find a significant increase in loneliness in 2020 that is not due to developmental processes of young adulthood but to imposed restriction of social interactions in the wake of the SARS-CoV-2 (COVID-19) pandemic (Buecker et al. 2020a).

In sum, both cross-sectional and longitudinal studies are associated with conceptual and practical strengths and limitations. With these caveats in mind, we now turn to the empirical evidence on loneliness across the life span.

Distribution of Loneliness Across the Life Span

A recent meta-analysis of longitudinal studies found a U-shaped trajectory such that average loneliness levels decrease during childhood, remain relatively stable across most of adulthood, and increase in old age (Mund et al. 2020a). These highly aggregated data reflect broad trends in the lifetime development of loneliness. For a more nuanced picture of trajectories within specific age groups, we now discuss single studies examining age differences and mean-level changes in loneliness from childhood to old age.

Most studies find that loneliness decreases during childhood (Harris et al. 2013; Hsieh and Yen 2019) and adolescence (Ladd and Ettekal 2013; Vanhalst et al. 2013). However, there are also substantial individual differences in these changes. One way to examine these differences is to use latent class modeling to identify distinct trajectories of loneliness (Harris et al. 2013; Qualter et al. 2013; Schinka et al. 2013). For example, in a five-wave, cohort-sequential longitudinal study of Dutch teenagers, 63% had stable low levels of loneliness, but 18% had high increasing loneliness, and 3% had permanently high levels of loneliness (Vanhalst et al. 2013). Thus, although childhood and adolescence are not generally characterized by increasing loneliness levels, sizable subgroups of children and adolescents do experience high or increasing levels of loneliness.

In addition, the observed trajectories might depend on how loneliness is measured. Most studies on loneliness in children and adolescents measure loneliness in specific contexts, such as school (Mund et al. 2020a; von Soest et al. 2020a) and therefore might provide an incomplete picture of these participants' loneliness experiences. In a study using longitudinal data from Norway (von Soest et al. 2020a), mean-level changes in loneliness were examined separately for emotional loneliness, social loneliness, and a direct single-item measure ("I feel lonely"). The estimated trajectories are depicted in Figure 3–1. Consistent with research focusing on loneliness in school, social loneliness decreased across adolescence and into young adulthood. Emotional loneliness and directly measured loneliness, in contrast, increased during adolescence until the mid-20s. A possible explanation for these divergent trajectories is that growing social networks (Wrzus et al. 2013) during this life phase protect against social loneliness but not against emotional loneliness. Emotional loneliness may be more strongly influenced by having close bonds that family members can no longer support as adolescents become more independent from their families (von Soest et al. 2020a).

Compared with childhood/adolescence and old age, studies examining changes in loneliness in mid-adulthood are scarce (Mund et al. 2020a) and

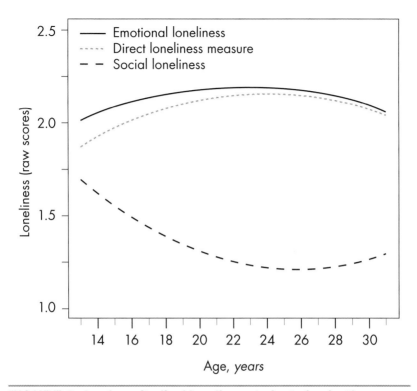

FIGURE 3–1. **Longitudinal loneliness trajectories for three measures of loneliness in a Norwegian sample.**

Source. Adapted from von Soest et al. 2020a.

provide a complicated picture. In some studies (Franssen et al. 2020; Hawkley et al. 2022; Luhmann and Hawkley 2016), loneliness levels tend to be elevated in midlife (approximately 40–60 years) (Figure 3–2). Others find the opposite pattern, with lower or decreasing loneliness levels in middle-aged adults than in young or older adults (Boomsma et al. 2007; Nicolaisen and Thorsen 2014).

The picture becomes more consistent again into older age. From midlife to old age, the trajectories typically follow a U-shaped form, such that loneliness levels decrease from mid-adulthood to early old age and then increase again, with the turning point around ages 70–75 years. This pattern has been found in both cross-sectional and longitudinal data from various countries including (in alphabetical order) China (Yang et al. 2018), Germany (Böger and Huxhold 2018a; Luhmann and Hawkley 2016), the Netherlands (Dykstra et al. 2005; Suanet and van Tilburg 2019; van Ours 2021), Norway (Nicolaisen and Thorsen 2014; von Soest et al. 2020b), the United

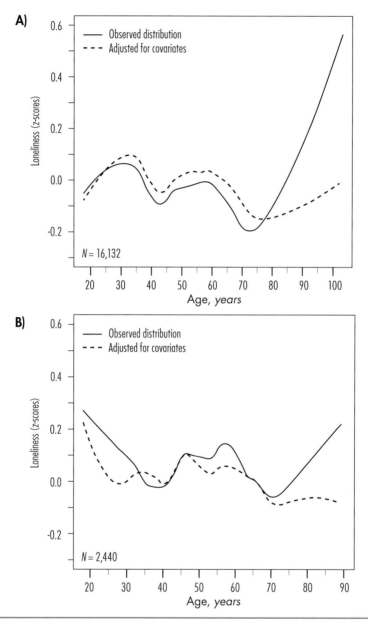

FIGURE 3–2.   **Cross-sectional age distribution in loneliness in the German Socioeconomic Panel Study (*A*) and the U.S. General Social Survey (*B*).**

Solid lines illustrate the observed age distribution. *Dashed lines* illustrate the distribution after adjusting for covariates such as marital status, health, or income. *Source.*   Panel A data from Luhmann and Hawkley 2016; Panel B data from Hawkley et al. 2022.

Kingdom (Victor and Yang 2012), and the United States (Hawkley and Kocherginsky 2018; Hawkley et al. 2019, 2022). Cross-national comparisons of European countries indicate that the late-life increase in loneliness is particularly pronounced in Southern (Dykstra 2009; Yang and Victor 2011) and Eastern European countries (Hansen and Slagsvold 2016) compared with Northern and Western European countries.

A substantial number of these studies are cross-sectional and provide a snapshot of the age distribution of loneliness at a particular point in time. As discussed earlier, the studies are mute on whether the observed age differences are due to age effects or cohort effects. Only a few studies so far have directly examined cohort differences in loneliness. The meta-analysis of longitudinal studies mentioned earlier did not find any significant generational differences in levels of loneliness (Mund et al. 2020a). Among older adults, some studies found higher loneliness levels among earlier-born cohorts than among later-born cohorts (Dykstra 2009; Hülür et al. 2016; Suanet and van Tilburg 2019), but this pattern was not replicated in all studies (Hawkley et al. 2019). Among emerging adults (ages 18–29 years), a recent meta-analysis found the opposite pattern, such that earlier-born cohorts had lower loneliness levels on average than later-born cohorts (Buecker et al. 2021b). Overall, there is no evidence that loneliness levels are generally increasing; rather, studies suggest that most of the age differences in loneliness can be explained by age effects rather than cohort effects (Hawkley et al. 2019; Suanet and van Tilburg 2019).

Robust empirical evidence has shown that loneliness tends to decrease through childhood and adolescence and to increase after about age 75. The evidence is less consistent with respect to middle adulthood, which is partly due to a lack of (longitudinal) studies focusing on this age period.

Predictors of Loneliness Across the Life Span

Age differences in loneliness can be due to age-related changes in the prevalence or relevance of predictors of loneliness. *Prevalence effects* mean that age differences in loneliness are due to an unequal distribution of risk factors in different age groups. Holding these risk factors constant (e.g., by including them as covariates in a regression model) should reduce the observed age differences in loneliness. *Relevance effects* mean that the relative impact of a predictor differs as a function by age. Relevance effects can be detected by examining the association between a specific predictor and loneliness separately in different age groups or, more elegantly, by testing the statistical interaction between this predictor and age. A significant interaction would indicate that the relative impact of a predictor on loneliness depends on age.

Although prevalence and relevance effects are rarely directly compared, the predominance of existing research suggests that most age differences in loneliness are due to age differences in the prevalence rather than the relevance of predictors. This is particularly the case for old age. In several studies, higher levels of loneliness among the oldest-old can be almost fully explained by a higher prevalence of poor physical health, widowhood, smaller social networks, and fewer social interactions (Aartsen and Jylhä 2011; Brittain et al. 2017; Cohen-Mansfield et al. 2013; Dahlberg et al. 2022; Hawkley et al. 2022; Luhmann and Hawkley 2016). Being unmarried was perhaps the most important factor accounting for higher loneliness in this age group (Brittain et al. 2017; Cohen-Mansfield et al. 2016; Dykstra et al. 2005). For example, take the age distributions depicted in Figure 3–2. In both studies, the high loneliness levels among the oldest-old almost completely disappear after adjusting for various covariates such as health or marital status. In addition, several studies found that for most established predictors, the strength of their association with loneliness did not differ significantly as a function of age (Hawkley et al. 2022; Luhmann and Hawkley 2016; von Soest et al. 2020b).

Nevertheless, for some predictors, age differences in their relevance for loneliness have been reported. With respect to personality, one meta-analysis found that the relationship between extraversion and loneliness was weaker and the relationship between openness to experiences and loneliness was stronger in samples with higher average age than in samples with lower average age (Buecker et al. 2020b). A meta-analysis on sex differences found that males were somewhat lonelier than females during childhood, adolescence, and young adulthood, but there were no significant sex differences in older age groups (Maes et al. 2019). Low income and less education tend to be risk factors for loneliness in all age groups, but the effect is less strong among older people (Franssen et al. 2020; Luhmann and Hawkley 2016; Yang et al. 2018). Similarly, being single is robustly associated with higher loneliness across the entire adult life span, but this effect is weaker among young adults up to age 30 (Child and Lawton 2019; Luhmann and Hawkley 2016) and again among older adults (Böger and Huxhold 2020; Yang et al. 2018) than among middle-aged adults.

The quantity (e.g., number of friends, size of the social network, contact frequency) and quality (e.g., having a close confidant, being satisfied with one's relationships) of one's social relationships are important predictors of loneliness across the life span. However, as mentioned, their relative importance changes with time, with quality becoming more important than quantity from childhood to adolescence and emerging adulthood (Qualter et al. 2015; von Soest et al. 2020a; Weeks and Asher 2012), throughout adulthood (Franssen et al. 2020), and up to old age (Nicolaisen and Thorsen 2014; Nyqvist et al. 2016; Pinquart and Sörensen 2003). This does not mean, however, that older people are indifferent to changes in the size of their social networks. In one study, increases in loneliness after widowhood were similar across age groups (Buecker et al. 2021a). Another study focusing on 40- to 80-year-old adults even found that loneliness increased more among older people than among middle-aged people after losses in one's social network (Böger and Huxhold 2018b), presumably because these network losses were more likely to be involuntary and irreversible in older than in younger people.

A relatively novel and particularly dynamic field of research concerns the impact of social media use on loneliness. Current research suggests that social media usage can be a protective factor if it supplements one's social interactions but a risk factor for loneliness if it replaces offline social interactions (Nowland et al. 2018). Older adults seem more likely to use social media in the former way, whereas adolescents and young adults are more likely to use social media in the latter way (Nowland et al. 2018).

We must emphasize that all of these findings on predictors of loneliness are based on studies conducted prior to the COVID-19 pandemic. The pandemic has led to increases in loneliness levels across all age groups (for a review, see Buecker and Horstmann 2021). At this time, it is unclear how loneliness levels in the general population and in different age groups will change once the pandemic is under control.

Outcomes of Loneliness Across the Life Span

Chronic loneliness is associated with poor mental and physical health outcomes and reduced life expectancy across the life span (for reviews, see Cacioppo and Cacioppo 2018; Hawkley and Capitanio 2015; Holt-Lunstad et al. 2015; see also Chapter 7, "Systemic Neuroendocrine and Inflammatory Mechanisms in Loneliness"). Age differences in these outcomes do not concern whether loneliness impairs health in general, but which health indicators are affected in specific age groups. For example, among older adults, chronic loneliness can lead to health issues that are generally more common in old age, such as diabetes or dementia (Hawkley and Capitanio 2015; Yang et al. 2016). In contrast, health issues that are not inherently age-related, such as sleep disorders, reduced physical activity, depressive symptoms, or poor immune functioning, have been associated with loneliness across the entire life span (Hawkley and Capitanio 2015; Yang et al.

2016). Importantly, experiences of loneliness during adolescence and young adulthood can have long-term consequences, such as poor health and lower income in midlife, and may lead to chronic diseases in older adulthood (Caspi et al. 2006; von Soest et al. 2020a). Because loneliness contributes to these outcomes, it must be addressed earlier in life, before disease-related physiological changes become irreversible. In sum, although most research on outcomes of loneliness has focused on older adults, loneliness can lead to adverse outcomes at any age.

Implications for Prevention and Intervention

Individual- and community-level interventions to prevent and reduce loneliness are often targeted at older adults (see Fakoya et al. 2020). Our review has shown that older adults are indeed the age group most at risk of experiencing loneliness, particularly those age 80 years and older. However, we also demonstrated that loneliness can occur and is associated with adverse health outcomes at any age. Hence, effective prevention and intervention are needed for all age groups.

People who feel lonely often avoid contact with others (Cacioppo and Cacioppo 2018; Qualter et al. 2015). This symptom of loneliness poses a challenge for prevention and intervention because one cannot expect lonely people to seek out help actively. It is therefore necessary to identify and reach those who are at risk of becoming lonely and those who already feel lonely. A first step is to define demographic groups that are particularly at risk. For older adults, these groups are already well-defined, thanks to the focus of previous research on this population. Among older adults, those who are unmarried and those who have recently been widowed are particularly at risk (Cohen-Mansfield et al. 2016). Among young and middle-aged adults, however, it is much harder to define specific demographic risk groups, partly due to a lack of research in these age groups. Of course, demographic characteristics are always an imperfect tool for identifying risk groups. Most widowed seniors are not lonely, and many who are lonely may not fall into one of these demographic groups. Nevertheless, defining demographic risk groups can be a good starting point to design interventions, particularly on the community level (see Chapter 10, "Community-Based Interventions for Loneliness").

Once risk groups are defined, they need to be reached. Here, age differences become very salient. Most people are online and can be reached by or actively search for online resources, social media campaigns, and social groups organized online. Among the very old, however, a significant number do not have access to online resources and often do not know to whom they should turn (see "Case Vignette: Mr. Sanchez" later). One promising approach for reaching lonely older adults is through their primary care provider. Educating primary care providers on recognizing loneliness in their patients and providing them with specific interventions (e.g., social prescribing in the United Kingdom) can be an effective way to reach and help lonely people. However, this approach probably works better for seniors than for younger adults who visit their primary care providers much less frequently.

Case Vignette: Mr. Sanchez

Mr. Sanchez was 95 years old when, for the first time in his life, he was alone at Christmas. His children lived far away and were not allowed to travel because of the COVID-19 pandemic, his wife had been dead for 2 years, and he lived alone. Feeling lonely and wanting to toast Christmas with someone, he came up with an unusual idea: he dialed 911. "Hello, there's nothing wrong with me, I just need someone to toast Christmas with. Would they have an officer who could stop by my house for a few minutes?" A little later, two police officers stopped by his house. The officers found Mr. Sanchez physically well and very happy to see someone. They stayed for over an hour, toasted Christmas, chatted about old times and listened to stories about Mr. Sanchez' experiences in World War II. After making a video call with him to his children, the officers had to leave because of an emergency but still had time to take a souvenir photo.

Finally, the intervention itself should be age-appropriate (see Chapter 8, "Interventions for Loneliness in Younger People," and Chapter 9, "Interventions for Loneliness in Older Adults"). In general, interventions aimed at reducing maladaptive cognitions appear to be effective in all age groups (Masi et al. 2011). Nevertheless, age differences in the prevalence and relevance of specific loneliness predictors should be considered in clinical interventions. For example, a young adult student who is single is in a different situation than a 90-year-old who is grieving the loss of their lifetime spouse (see "Case Vignette: Angela"). Both may experience intense loneliness, but the specific causes of their loneliness and their control over these causes are very different. Finding a partner is a realistic and attainable goal for a young adult, so this person would probably benefit most from an intervention that gives them the confidence to connect with other like-minded singles. In contrast, the bereaved senior presumably would not be very interested in signing up for speed dating nights but would rather benefit from an intervention helping them come to terms with the loss of their spouse. These examples may be simplistic, but they illustrate how age-dependent causes of loneliness must be considered when designing loneliness interventions.

Moreover, the efficacy of specific interventions may differ between age groups, so both individual-level and community-level interventions need to be evaluated separately in different age groups (Bessaha et al. 2020; Eccles and Qualter 2021; Fakoya et al. 2020).

Case Vignette: Angela

Angela has known loneliness for almost all of her life. Her parents have always described her as somewhat reserved and cautious. When Angela started school, she was initially unaccustomed to being among so many children and was afraid of the noise and unpredictable wildness of the other children. As time went on, however, she gained confidence; a good relationship with her teacher helped her a lot. When she moved on to secondary school, she again needed time to build up trust with the new teachers and children but eventually got on well there and even found a friend with whom she often met at home.

At the age of 12, her friend left the school, and a new student joined the class. This new student quickly realized that Angela could not defend herself well against jokes at her expense and increasingly made her a target. As Angela became increasingly withdrawn, irritable, and anxious, her parents took notice and realized that their daughter was a victim of bullying. When discussions with the teachers did not bring about a fundamental change, they transferred Angela to another school. At the new school, Angela was safe from the attacks by her tormentor, but she had little trust in her classmates and teachers. She felt increasingly lonely. In addition, she had doubts about her appearance and the physical changes with puberty. Other girls seemed to have much fewer problems than her, and some even reported experiences with boys and talked about alcohol and drugs. Angela increasingly perceived herself as an outsider and a freak. This only changed for the better when she met a new classmate, Nicole, with whom she became lifelong friends.

Angela met her boyfriend, Tom, at college. After graduation, they both started a job in a large and expensive city and moved there together. They both met many people at work, but because they frequently moved between different clients, often working longer hours in different locations with little time for leisure, they did not develop any real close relationships. Luckily, they were on the same team. Over time, however, their relationship became strained. Tom started a new job that required him to travel a lot. Angela missed their regular contact and often felt lonely. She particularly missed the opportunity to have someone with whom to share her emotions and her less obvious interests in contemporary art and European cinema. It was no fun to go to exhibitions and movies alone, and she definitely did not dine out alone. Her friend Nicole was far away and was busy with her children and her own job. Angela had not found a real substitute, and the phone and video calls with Nicole were not really satisfying. Tom accused Angela of being too clingy and suggested she do something with other people, but she did not dare because she felt bored and often inadequate in company.

Shortly after Angela's 36th birthday, Tom left her for a colleague at his job, and her world collapsed. Although her work at the office was appreciated, she was alone there for a large part of the time. She had long experienced the big city as anonymous, unfriendly, and even downright threatening. She longed for someone with whom she could communicate without fear but did not know how to meet such a person. She increasingly stayed alone, not only during breaks at work but also at home in the evenings and on weekends. She soon slipped into a downward spiral of passive withdrawal, lack of positive experiences, and emotional isolation. When she learned that Tom's new partner was now expecting his child, she felt completely depressed and worthless, as though she had no strength left for anything.

A psychiatrist diagnosed Angela with major depressive disorder and prescribed a selective serotonin reuptake inhibitor, as well as a benzodiazepine for her sleep problems and rumination. The medication helped her sleep, but it was not very restful; she continued to feel unable to get up for anything and struggled at work. When she tried to sleep without the benzodiazepine, she had panic attacks and felt "totally miserable," so she continued to take it, which further undermined her self-worth and self-efficacy. Shortly thereafter, she read an article that said many people taking antidepressants cannot quit. Worried, she decided to make a new discontinuation attempt with a clinical psychologist.

The clinical psychologist diagnosed Angela with social anxiety disorder with comorbid major depressive disorder and referred her, through a social worker, to an art club that visited a gallery of contemporary art or an exhibition every week in small groups of five or six people and often with an art historian who commented on the works. This social activity gave her a structure and a new circle of acquaintances with interests similar to hers and soon became an important part of her free time. At the same time, the therapist helped her slowly overcome her distorted negative view of herself. Specific self-confidence exercises and social skills training were also a great help. Above all, however, the art club helped her; as she put it later, "art has saved my life." Angela no longer felt so lonely and had renewed confidence because she experienced that she was able to make meaningful connections with people with whom she shared a deep common interest. She decided never to let herself go like that again.

Summary

In this chapter, we reviewed the theoretical and empirical research on loneliness across the life span. Despite being a relatively stable construct, loneliness can and does change over time. Both cross-sectional and longitudinal studies indicate that loneliness tends to decrease during childhood and adolescence and to increase in old age, particularly after age 80. The development of loneliness during mid-adulthood is less well known due to a lack of studies focusing on this age period.

Age differences in loneliness can be explained by age differences in the prevalence and relevance of risk factors. In old age, risk factors such as widowhood, social isolation, and functional limitations become more prevalent and can explain the elevated loneliness levels in this population. With time, the quantity of those social relationships becomes less important and the quality of one's social relationships becomes more important. These age differences in the relevance of certain risk factors have important implications for preventing and combating loneliness. Strategies aimed at identifying and reaching lonely people and interventions targeted at reducing loneliness must be age-appropriate.

KEY POINTS

- Older people are particularly at risk of feeling lonely because widowhood, social isolation, and functional limitations due to poor health are more common in this age group.

- Loneliness can occur at any age.

- Interventions for reducing loneliness should be age-appropriate.

- Younger people may benefit more from interventions aimed at establishing opportunities for social interactions and improving their social skills than older adults.

Suggested Readings

Hawkley LC, Capitanio JP: Perceived social isolation, evolutionary fitness and health outcomes: a lifespan approach. Philos Trans R Soc Lond B Biol Sci 370(1669):20140114, 2015 25870400

Luhmann M, Hawkley LC: Age differences in loneliness from late adolescence to oldest old age. Dev Psychol 52(6):943–959, 2016 27148782

Mund M, Freuding MM, Möbius K, et al: The stability and change of loneliness across the life span: a meta-analysis of longitudinal studies. Pers Soc Psychol Rev 24(1):24–52, 2020

Qualter P, Vanhalst J, Harris R, et al: Loneliness across the life span. Perspect Psychol Sci 10(2):250–264, 2015 25910393

von Soest T, Luhmann M, Gerstorf D: The development of loneliness through adolescence and young adulthood: its nature, correlates, and midlife outcomes. Dev Psychol 56(10):1919–1934, 2020

References

Aartsen M, Jylhä M: Onset of loneliness in older adults: results of a 28 year prospective study. Eur J Ageing 8(1):31–38, 2011 21475393

Asher SR, Paquette JA: Loneliness and peer relations in childhood. Curr Dir Psychol Sci 12(3):75–78, 2003

Baumeister RF, Leary MR: The need to belong: desire for interpersonal attachments as a fundamental human motivation. Psychol Bull 117(3):497–529, 1995 7777651

Bessaha ML, Sabbath EL, Morris Z, et al: A systematic review of loneliness interventions among non-elderly adults. Clin Soc Work J 48(1):110–125, 2020

Böger A, Huxhold O: Age-related changes in emotional qualities of the social network from middle adulthood into old age: how do they relate to the experience of loneliness? Psychol Aging 33(3):482–496, 2018a 29446969

Böger A, Huxhold O: Do the antecedents and consequences of loneliness change from middle adulthood into old age? Dev Psychol 54(1):181–197, 2018b 29154641

Böger A, Huxhold O: The changing relationship between partnership status and loneliness: effects related to aging and historical time. J Gerontol B Psychol Sci Soc Sci 75(7):1423–1432, 2020 30590817

Boomsma DI, Cacioppo JT, Muthén B, et al: Longitudinal genetic analysis for loneliness in Dutch twins. Twin Res Hum Genet 10(2):267–273, 2007 17564516

Borys S, Perlman D: Gender differences in loneliness. Pers Soc Psychol Bull 11(1):63–74, 1985

Brittain K, Kingston A, Davies K, et al: An investigation into the patterns of loneliness and loss in the oldest old: Newcastle 85+ Study. Ageing Soc 37(1):39–62, 2017

Buecker S, Horstmann KT: Loneliness and social isolation during the COVID-19 pandemic: a systematic review enriched with empirical evidence from a large-scale diary study. Unpublished manuscript, 2021

Buecker S, Horstmann KT, Krasko J, et al: Changes in daily loneliness for German residents during the first four weeks of the COVID-19 pandemic. Soc Sci Med 265:113541, 2020a 33248868

Buecker S, Maes M, Denissen JJA, Luhmann M: Loneliness and the big five personality traits: a meta–analysis. Eur J Pers 34(1):8–28, 2020b

Buecker S, Denissen JJA, Luhmann M: A propensity-score matched study of changes in loneliness surrounding major life events. J Pers Soc Psychol 121(3):669–690, 2021a 33119390

Buecker S, Mund M, Chwastek S, et al: Is loneliness in emerging adults increasing over time? A preregistered cross-temporal meta-analysis and systematic review. Psychol Bull 147(8):787–805, 2021b

Cacioppo JT, Cacioppo S: Loneliness in the modern age: an evolutionary theory of loneliness (ETL). Adv Exp Soc Psychol 58:127–197, 2018

Carmichael CL, Reis HT, Duberstein PR: In your 20s it's quantity, in your 30s it's quality: the prognostic value of social activity across 30 years of adulthood. Psychol Aging 30(1):95–105, 2015 25774426

Carstensen LL, Isaacowitz DM, Charles ST: Taking time seriously: a theory of socioemotional selectivity. Am Psychol 54(3):165–181, 1999 10199217

Caspi A, Harrington H, Moffitt TE, et al: Socially isolated children 20 years later: risk of cardiovascular disease. Arch Pediatr Adolesc Med 160(8):805–811, 2006 16894079

Child ST, Lawton L: Loneliness and social isolation among young and late middle-age adults: associations with personal networks and social participation. Aging Ment Health 23(2):196–204, 2019 29171764

Cohen-Mansfield J, Shmotkin D, Blumstein Z, et al: The old, old-old, and the oldest old: continuation or distinct categories? An examination of the relationship between age and changes in health, function, and wellbeing. Int J Aging Hum Dev 77(1):37–57, 2013 23986979

Cohen-Mansfield J, Hazan H, Lerman Y, Shalom V: Correlates and predictors of loneliness in older-adults: a review of quantitative results informed by qualitative insights. Int Psychogeriatr 28(4):557–576, 2016 26424033

Dahlberg L, McKee KJ, Frank A, Naseer M: A systematic review of longitudinal risk factors for loneliness in older adults. Aging Ment Health 26:225–249, 2022 33563024

Danneel S, Maes M, Bijttebier P, et al: Loneliness and attitudes toward aloneness in Belgian adolescents: measurement invariance across language, age, and gender groups. J Psychopathol Behav Assess 40(4):678–690, 2018

De Jong Gierveld J, van Tilburg T: A 6-item scale for overall, emotional, and social loneliness. Res Aging 28(5):582–598, 2006

Dykstra PA: Older adult loneliness: myths and realities. Eur J Ageing 6(2):91–100, 2009 19517025

Dykstra PA, van Tilburg TG, de Jong Gierveld J: Changes in older adult loneliness. Res Aging 27(6):725–747, 2005

Eccles AM, Qualter P: Alleviating loneliness in young people: a meta-analysis of interventions. Child Adolesc Ment Health 26(1):17–33, 2021 32406165

Fakoya OA, McCorry NK, Donnelly M: Loneliness and social isolation interventions for older adults: a scoping review of reviews. BMC Public Health 20(1):129, 2020 32054474

Franssen T, Stijnen M, Hamers F, Schneider F: Age differences in demographic, social and health-related factors associated with loneliness across the adult life span (19–65 years): a cross-sectional study in the Netherlands. BMC Public Health 20(1):1118, 2020 32758200

Goossens L, van Roekel E, Verhagen M, et al: The genetics of loneliness: linking evolutionary theory to genome-wide genetics, epigenetics, and social science. Perspect Psychol Sci 10(2):213–226, 2015 25910391

Hansen T, Slagsvold B: Late-life loneliness in 11 European countries: results from the Generations and Gender Survey. Soc Indic Res 129(1):445–464, 2016

Harris RA, Qualter P, Robinson SJ: Loneliness trajectories from middle childhood to pre-adolescence: impact on perceived health and sleep disturbance. J Adolesc 36(6):1295–1304, 2013 23403089

Hawkley LC, Cacioppo JT: Aging and loneliness. Curr Dir Psychol Sci 16(4):187–191, 2007

Hawkley LC, Capitanio JP: Perceived social isolation, evolutionary fitness and health outcomes: a lifespan approach. Philos Trans R Soc Lond B Biol Sci 370(1669):20140114, 2015 25870400

Hawkley LC, Kocherginsky M: Transitions in loneliness among older adults: a 5-year follow-up in the National Social Life, Health, and Aging Project. Res Aging 40(4):365–387, 2018 29519211

Hawkley LC, Wroblewski K, Kaiser T, et al: Are U.S. older adults getting lonelier? Age, period, and cohort differences. Psychol Aging 34(8):1144–1157, 2019 31804118

Hawkley LC, Buecker S, Kaiser T, Luhmann M: Loneliness from young adulthood to old age: explaining age differences in loneliness. Int J Behav Dev 46:39–49, 2022 35001993

Heckhausen J, Wrosch C, Schulz R: A motivational theory of life-span development. Psychol Rev 117(1):32–60, 2010 20063963

Holt-Lunstad J, Smith TB, Baker M, et al: Loneliness and social isolation as risk factors for mortality: a meta-analytic review. Perspect Psychol Sci 10(2):227–237, 2015 25910392

Hsieh Y-P, Yen L-L: Trajectories of loneliness and aggression from childhood to early adolescence in Taiwan: the roles of parenting and demographic predictors. J Early Adolesc 39(3):313–339, 2019

Hülür G, Drewelies J, Eibich P, et al: Cohort differences in psychosocial function over 20 years: current older adults feel less lonely and less dependent on external circumstances. Gerontology 62(3):354–361, 2016 26820135

Ladd GW, Ettekal I: Peer-related loneliness across early to late adolescence: normative trends, intra-individual trajectories, and links with depressive symptoms. J Adolesc 36(6):1269–1282, 2013 23787076

Luhmann M, Hawkley LC: Age differences in loneliness from late adolescence to oldest old age. Dev Psychol 52(6):943–959, 2016 27148782

Maes M, Klimstra T, van den Noortgate W, Goossens L: Factor structure and measurement invariance of a multidimensional loneliness scale: comparisons across gender and age. J Child Fam Stud 24(6):1829–1837, 2015

Maes M, Qualter P, Vanhalst J, et al: Gender differences in loneliness across the lifespan: a meta–analysis. Eur J Pers 33(6):642–654, 2019

Masi CM, Chen H-Y, Hawkley LC, Cacioppo JT: A meta-analysis of interventions to reduce loneliness. Pers Soc Psychol Rev 15(3):219–266, 2011 20716644

Merz E-M, Jak S: The long reach of childhood. Childhood experiences influence close relationships and loneliness across life. Adv Life Course Res 18(3):212–222, 2013 24796560

Mund M, Freuding MM, Möbius K, et al: The stability and change of loneliness across the life span: a meta-analysis of longitudinal studies. Pers Soc Psychol Rev 24(1):24–52, 2020a 31179872

Mund M, Lüdtke O, Neyer FJ: Owner of a lonely heart: the stability of loneliness across the life span. J Pers Soc Psychol 119(2):497–516, 2020b 31556683

Nicolaisen M, Thorsen K: Who are lonely? Loneliness in different age groups (18–81 years old), using two measures of loneliness. Int J Aging Hum Dev 78(3):229–257, 2014 25265679

Nowland R, Necka EA, Cacioppo JT: Loneliness and social internet use: pathways to reconnection in a digital world? Perspect Psychol Sci 13(1):70–87, 2018 28937910

Nyqvist F, Victor CR, Forsman AK, Cattan M: The association between social capital and loneliness in different age groups: a population-based study in Western Finland. BMC Public Health 16:542, 2016 27400659

Peplau LA, Perlman D (eds): Loneliness: A Sourcebook of Current Theory, Research, and Therapy. Hoboken, NJ, Wiley Interscience, 1982

Pinquart M, Sörensen S: Risk factors for loneliness in adulthood and old age: a meta-analysis, in Advances in Psychology Research, Vol 19. Edited by Shohov SP. Hauppauge, NY, Nova Science Publishers, 2003, pp 111–143

Qualter P, Brown SL, Rotenberg KJ, et al: Trajectories of loneliness during childhood and adolescence: predictors and health outcomes. J Adolesc 36(6):1283–1293, 2013 23465384

Qualter P, Vanhalst J, Harris R, et al: Loneliness across the life span. Perspect Psychol Sci 10(2):250–264, 2015 25910393

Russell DW: UCLA Loneliness Scale (Version 3): reliability, validity, and factor structure. J Pers Assess 66(1):20–40, 1996 8576833

Sander J, Schupp J, Richter D: Getting together: social contact frequency across the life span. Dev Psychol 53(8):1571–1588, 2017 28541063

Schinka KC, van Dulmen MHM, Mata AD, et al: Psychosocial predictors and outcomes of loneliness trajectories from childhood to early adolescence. J Adolesc 36(6):1251–1260, 2013 24007942

Suanet B, van Tilburg TG: Loneliness declines across birth cohorts: the impact of mastery and self-efficacy. Psychol Aging 34(8):1134–1143, 2019 31804117

van Ours JC: What a drag it is getting old? Mental health and loneliness beyond age 50. Appl Econ 53:3563–3576, 2021

Vanhalst J, Goossens L, Luyckx K, et al: The development of loneliness from mid- to late adolescence: trajectory classes, personality traits, and psychosocial functioning. J Adolesc 36(6):1305–1312, 2013 22560517

Victor CR, Yang K: The prevalence of loneliness among adults: a case study of the United Kingdom. J Psychol 146(1–2):85–104, 2012 22303614

von Soest T, Luhmann M, Gerstorf D: The development of loneliness through adolescence and young adulthood: its nature, correlates, and midlife outcomes. Dev Psychol 56(10):1919–1934, 2020a 32852969

von Soest T, Luhmann M, Hansen T, Gerstorf D: Development of loneliness in midlife and old age: its nature and correlates. J Pers Soc Psychol 118(2):388–406, 2020b 30284871

Weeks MS, Asher SR: Loneliness in childhood: toward the next generation of assessment and research. Adv Child Dev Behav 42:1–39, 2012

Wrzus C, Hänel M, Wagner J, Neyer FJ: Social network changes and life events across the life span: a meta-analysis. Psychol Bull 139(1):53–80, 2013 22642230

Yang F, Zhang J, Wang J: Correlates of loneliness in older adults in Shanghai, China: does age matter? BMC Geriatr 18(1):300, 2018 30509209

Yang K, Victor CR: Age and loneliness in 25 European nations. Ageing Soc 31(8):1368–1388, 2011

Yang YC, Boen C, Gerken K, et al: Social relationships and physiological determinants of longevity across the human life span. Proc Natl Acad Sci USA 113(3):578–583, 2016 26729882

4

Loneliness in People Living With Mental Health Disorders

Miya M. Gentry, M.A.
Barton W. Palmer, Ph.D.

THE PRESENCE OF LONELINESS in the context of mental disorders warrants special attention in clinical care and research. Although the prevalence of loneliness in the general population is of notable concern, the rates among persons living with mental health disorders are even higher, including estimates as high as 80% among people with schizophrenia (Stain et al. 2012). Loneliness is also highly prevalent among people presenting to mental health crisis centers (Wang et al. 2019). The significance of these figures rests not only in the aversive nature of loneliness but also in its adverse effects on physiological functioning, cognitive and physical health, well-being, and mortality (Holt-Lunstad 2021; National Academies of Sci-

This work was supported in part by National Institute of Mental Health grant R01MH120201 and by the Department of Veterans Affairs. The authors have no conflicts to disclose. The contents do not represent the views of the U.S. Department of Veterans Affairs or the U.S. government.

ences, Engineering, and Medicine 2020; see also Chapter 7 "Systemic Neuroendocrine and Inflammatory Mechanisms in Loneliness"). Loneliness is also a risk factor for suicidal ideation and behavior.

The goal of this chapter is to provide an overview of the current empirical literature on loneliness in people living with mental health disorders and to provide information and suggestions applicable to provisions of clinical care. As we discuss, there are many gaps in the empirical data on loneliness and its prevention and treatment among people with serious mental illnesses, but there are already sufficient data to support direct clinical attention to loneliness and social isolation in mental health care settings. We start with a discussion of the general conceptual framework of the nature and meaning of loneliness and social isolation, with an emphasis on relevance to mental health care. We then discuss the available empirical literature on loneliness in the context of mental health disorders, including depression, bipolar disorder, anxiety, schizophrenia, and PTSD, and, where possible, comment on the clinical application of this information. Following this overview, we turn to recommendations for incorporating systematic assessment and treatment of loneliness in the context of mental health care. We conclude with two clinical vignettes to illustrate application of these considerations and recommendations.

General Framework

Why Is It Important to Consider Loneliness in People With Mental Health Concerns?

As noted elsewhere in this volume, the term *loneliness* refers to a distressing internal feeling resulting from a self-perceived discrepancy between the type, quality, or quantity of one's desired social relationships and network and the self-perceptions of one's actual social relationships and network. The capacity to feel loneliness appears to have been favored in human evolution through natural selection; research has shown it is moderately heritable ($h^2 = 0.37–0.44$) (Goossens et al. 2015; Spithoven et al. 2019; see also Chapter 2 "Loneliness, Other Aspects of Social Connection, and Their Measurement"). Analogous to the impact of acute versus chronic pain or hunger, however, there is a critical distinction between acute and chronic loneliness (Cacioppo and Hawkley 2005; Cacioppo and Patrick 2008).

According to the prevailing social neuroscience model of loneliness (Cacioppo and Hawkley 2005; Cacioppo and Patrick 2008), *acute loneliness* is a social drive that motivates individuals to seek social connections that may have benefits in terms of food, safety, and reproduction. In contrast, *chronic loneliness* may become biologically and socially toxic. This model has multiple components related to the initiation and maintenance of chronic loneliness and its downstream effects. A streamlined summary includes the following sequence: loneliness → hypervigilance to social safety concerns, social threat/cognitive biases (e.g., expecting and perceiving social interactions as negative) → negative social responses from others (resulting in snowball effect, acute loneliness becoming chronic loneliness) → feelings of stress, hostility, pessimism, anxiety, and low self-esteem → sustained physiological hyperarousal → adverse health outcomes and reduced well-being.

Physiological responses that are adaptive as short-term responses to threat become maladaptive when they are chronically activated, including dysregulation of key functions such as inflammatory and other immune responses, blood pressure, and metabolic function, thereby elevating risk for medical comorbidity. Many of the same physiological disruptions, medical comorbidities, and other downstream health outcomes associated with loneliness have also been implicated as contributing to accelerated biological aging in serious mental illnesses. Thus, chronic loneliness in the context of living with mental illness may represent a "double-hit" in terms of associated physical health outcomes.

Social Isolation Versus Loneliness

In the clinical care of people with mental health concerns, it is important to consider the distinction between loneliness and social isolation because each may warrant attention due to independent effects on health and mental and physical well-being. Although the relevant literature has been hampered by inconsistencies in terminology, in this chapter, we use the term *social isolation* in reference to the objectively quantifiable state of a person's social environment and relationships, such as frequency of social interactions and social network size, noting that these are usually measured using self-report (National Academies of Sciences, Engineering, and Medicine 2020). Loneliness and social isolation have a bidirectional relationship but are only modestly correlated ($r=0.20–0.30$) (Cornwell and Waite 2009; Green et al. 2018).

Phenomenological Experience of Loneliness and Mental Health Symptoms

As noted by Cacioppo et al. (2015), the perceived discrepancy between one's existing and one's desired social relationships "leads to the negative experience of feeling alone and/or the distress and dysphoria of feeling socially isolated even when among family or friends" (p. 238). Two words in this quote that stand out when considered in the context of mental health are *distress* and *dysphoria*. Psychological distress can take multiple forms; a partial list relevant to loneliness includes fear/anxiety, sadness, depressed mood, and irritability or resentment. The internal emotional experience of loneliness is best characterized as a "fuzzy set," with no single form of conscious distress being a required component of loneliness. One individual's conscious reaction to a self-perceived discrepancy in desired versus manifest social relationships may be sadness or depression, whereas in another individual anxiety about these perceived deficits may be most prominent. It can sometimes be challenging to establish a causal relationship between a primary mental health disorder such as depression and secondary feelings of loneliness.

Another critical component of the definition of *loneliness* is that the discrepancy is based in part on *self-perceptions* of one's actual social environment. Negative attribution biases of social cues and distortions in perceptions or beliefs about one's social isolation/connectedness can contribute to the development and persistence of loneliness but are also a core component of some forms of depression and anxiety. Addressing such maladaptive beliefs and cognitions is a key component of cognitive and cognitive-behavioral therapies.

Loneliness in Specific Mental Health Disorders

In this section we consider the relationship of loneliness to several mental health diagnoses. Some of these subsections are more detailed than others, in part reflecting the relative amount of empirical evidence available. As is noted, some concerns may be specific to the individual disorders, whereas others may be relevant to two or more conditions.

Depression

The association of loneliness and depression is complex. Empirical studies suggest that, relative to the general population, people with mood (or anxiety) disorders are more likely to report negative social relationships, social isolation, and feelings of loneliness. There appears to be a bidirectional, causal relationship, because loneliness may also result in increased social isolation and higher rates of depression across time. Recent data suggest that reducing loneliness could result in the prevention of 11%–18% of cases of depression in the population (Lee et al. 2021). Due to the frequent co-occurrence of depression and loneliness, some suggestions were made in the early 1970s to distinguish "lonely depressed" from "lonely not depressed" subtypes, but that typology has not been retained (Rook 1984).

One common misconception is that loneliness is just a symptom of depression rather than an independent entity. Although symptom scales for loneliness and depression are correlated with a moderate effect size of approximately $r=0.50$ (Erzen and Çikrikci 2018), factor analytic studies and other empirical data support the discriminant validity of these two constructs (Adams et al. 2004; Cacioppo et al. 2006; Russell et al. 1980; Weeks et al. 1980). Of particular relevance to clinical care is that loneliness and depression have independent effects on mortality risk (Holwerda et al. 2016; Rico-Uribe et al. 2018; Stek et al. 2005). The mechanisms by which loneliness may affect mortality beyond the effects of depression have been less thoroughly investigated, but even after adjusting for the effects of depression, loneliness has a significant adverse effect on biological markers of health and health outcomes, such as cardiovascular disease and dementia (Hawkley et al. 2006; Holwerda et al. 2014). There are also some preliminary data suggesting that loneliness and depression may be served by different underlying brain networks (Shao et al. 2020).

The clinical implications of the existing research are clear. Loneliness and depression are not synonymous, but they frequently co-occur and can potentiate each other. Thus, attention to both is essential when working with patients with depression or those presenting with loneliness or social isolation. One important consideration regarding loneliness among people with depression is the effect of depressive thought patterns on social relationships. Because of cognitive biases in depression, social interactions can be perceived as less gratifying and evaluated less favorably (National Academies of Sciences, Engineering, and Medicine 2020). This may increase social isolation and loneliness, further potentiating depressive symptoms. Breaking this cycle by addressing maladaptive cognitive patterns can be critical for clinical interventions.

Bipolar Disorders

Our recent search of the literature revealed surprisingly few empirical studies focused on loneliness among people with bipolar disorders. Given the predominance of depressive episodes typically experienced by people with a bipolar disorder and the frequent presence of residual depressive symptoms during inter-episode ("euthymic") periods, the considerations described for unipolar depression may equally apply to those with bipolar disorder. There is also evidence of inter-episode deficits in social cognitive functions among people with bipolar disorder that impact quality of social functioning (de Siqueira Rotenberg et al. 2020). Furthermore, disruptions in social relationships and social support may be triggered by specific behaviors present during manic or hypomanic episodes, such as impulsivity, increased sexual activity, reckless or risky behavior, and irritability. As with other mental health disorders, these relationships can be bidirectional because social support can also affect the long-term course and severity of bipolar disorder (Owen et al. 2017; Warren et al. 2018).

There has also been relevant research on the effects of bipolar disorder on married or other couples. One such study found that in couples in which one partner had bipolar disorder, the partner with bipolar disorder reported feelings of loneliness, shame, and helplessness (Granek et al. 2016). There is also a higher divorce rate among married couples in which one partner has a diagnosis of bipolar disorder (Grover et al. 2017).

There is a need for greater understanding of the temporal relationships between psychiatric symptoms, social isolation, and loneliness. Although it did not include a measure of loneliness, a study from our research group illustrated a viable approach to examining these temporal relationship (Kamarsu et al. 2020). Outpatients in this study with bipolar I or II disorder were administered twice-daily surveys of social activity and mood/affect and were followed for 11 weeks as part of a mobile device–delivered intervention study that used ecological momentary assessment. Lagged models indicated that greater social activity predicted better mood, but not the converse.

The relationship of manic/hypomanic and depressive symptoms and behaviors to loneliness and (healthy) social functioning may be helpful in clinical evaluations in individual therapy settings as well as in couples, family, or group therapies.

Anxiety Disorders

Despite limited epidemiological data on the prevalence of loneliness among people with anxiety disorders, these disorders appear to be strongly related to loneliness and social isolation. Social anxiety, generalized anxiety, panic disorder, and agoraphobia may all lead to behaviors that result in a narrowing of the social environment and increased loneliness. Individuals with anxiety disorders may intentionally narrow or retreat from their social networks due to the discomfort of social interactions or the anticipatory anxiety of such interactions. This narrowing of one's social network is consistent with the snowball effect/feedback loop model of persistent loneliness described by Cacioppo and colleagues (Cacioppo and Hawkley 2005; Cacioppo and Patrick 2008; Cacioppo et al. 2015).

Persistently lonely people become hyperattentive to cues of social rejection or social threat, resulting in further withdrawal and greater loneliness. Certain anxiety disorder factors may contribute to avoidance or withdrawal, including self-perceived stigma, fear of critical judgment or rejection, fear that others will notice and harshly judge the person's anxiety, and panic attacks triggered by social stimuli. Longitudinal research in the general population has documented a bidirectional temporal relationship between loneliness and social isolation over a 6-month follow-up period (Lim et al. 2016). Data in older adult samples also have indicated bidirectional effects of loneliness on generalized anxiety disorder or social anxiety disorder over a 2-year follow-up period (Domènech-Abella et al. 2019).

The clinical implications of the interaction of loneliness and anxiety are similar to those described earlier for depression. Not all anxious people are lonely, and not all lonely people are anxious, but there are strong bidirectional effects. Loneliness and anxiety are related forms of distress that have deleterious effects on physiological function and health outcomes. Thus, it is important to evaluate and address loneliness in patients presenting with anxiety and anxiety in patients presenting with loneliness.

Schizophrenia and Related Psychoses

Research attention to loneliness among people living with schizophrenia has increased in recent years. Studies of the prevalence of loneliness among people with schizophrenia suggest alarmingly high rates, ranging from 43% to 80% (Badcock et al. 2015; Beebe 2010; Eglit et al. 2018; Stain et al. 2012). Although not restricted to people with schizophrenia, meta-analyses have found small to medium associations between loneliness and the positive and negative symptoms of psychosis (Chau et al. 2019; Michalska da Rocha et al. 2018). Abdellaoui et al. (2018) showed that polygenic risk scores for schizophrenia predicted loneliness, even after controlling for risk of depression. A study from our research group found that the factor structure of items from the UCLA Loneliness Scale, Version 3 (UCLA LS3) was comparable among people living with schizophrenia and psychiatrically healthy comparison subjects (Eglit et al. 2018). The latter is consistent with the view that the construct of loneliness remains similar in people with schizophrenia relative to the general population.

The high prevalence of loneliness in schizophrenia may seem to be in conflict with *social anhedonia*, which characterizes some of the negative symptoms of schizophrenia. However, social anhedonia in schizophrenia is complex. There is a need to distinguish between a lack of social drive and a "learned helplessness" response to negative outcomes from others when trying to make social connections. This also relates to studies from clinical neuroscience on anticipatory versus experienced reward among people with schizophrenia. In other forms of reward, people with schizophrenia, on average, show deficits in anticipatory pleasure but not in experienced pleasure relative to psychiatrically healthy comparison subjects (Gard et al. 2007). It is unknown whether this pattern generalizes to anticipatory versus experienced pleasure from social interactions.

Loneliness has been identified as a high priority by people with schizophrenia and their supporters (Fortuna et al. 2019; Shumway et al. 2004), and it is significantly (negatively) related to personal sense of recovery among people with this disorder (Roe et al. 2011). Thirty-seven percent of adults with psychoses in a large-scale Australian survey identified loneliness as one of their most significant challenges (Morgan et al. 2017). Similar perceptions of loneliness as a priority have been found in qualitative studies of people living with schizophrenia (Beebe 2010; Davidson and Stayner 1997). Loneliness has also been shown to be associated with higher health care utilization among people with psychosis (Badcock et al. 2020). There is also a strong correlation between loneliness and self-perceived stigma among people with schizophrenia (Yildirim and Kavak Budak 2020), which is also consistent with Cacioppo and colleagues' model of social cognitive factors that contribute to persistent loneliness.

Schizophrenia itself is a risk factor for many of the same health outcomes and medical comorbidities that are related to loneliness. Due to the frequency of age-related medical comorbidities among people with schizophrenia, some researchers conceptualize it as a systemic disorder resulting in accelerated biological aging. Given the high prevalence of loneliness among people with schizophrenia, it is possible that some of the proximal causes of accelerated aging in schizophrenia could be attributable to social isolation and loneliness. Large-scale research to examine this possibility are ongoing, but published research at present is insufficient for drawing definitive conclusions.

Loneliness is rarely evaluated or targeted for treatment in routine mental health care for people with schizophrenia, despite its high prevalence, its implications for health and well-being, and its frequent description as a priority among people with schizophrenia and their families or caregivers. Although there have been a few promising feasibility studies (Lim et al. 2020a, 2020b) and multiple studies focused on social skills training and maladaptive thinking, there is a paucity of intervention studies addressing loneliness among people with schizophrenia or related disorders.

Posttraumatic Stress Disorder

The deleterious impact of PTSD on social functioning has been well documented, as has the potential positive effect of social support on the course and severity of PTSD. Many of the cardinal symptoms of PTSD have obvious relevance to social functioning, including feelings of detachment from others, avoidance behaviors, irritability, and hypervigilance. Despite this relevance to PTSD, there is a surprising dearth of empirical research on loneliness in PTSD. However, some studies have documented an association between trauma exposure, *symptoms* of PTSD, and loneliness. For example, loneliness is higher in veterans with PTSD symptoms than among those without PTSD symptoms (Kuwert et al. 2014). van der Velden et al. (2018) found that among people who have experienced a recent trauma, those reporting symptoms of PTSD also reported higher levels of loneliness than those with minimal or no PTSD symptoms. Furthermore, in a large longitudinal population survey from Amsterdam, Fox et al. (2021) found that changes in loneliness were (positively) associated with changes in PTSD symptoms.

Solomon and colleagues (Itzhaky et al. 2017; Solomon and Dekel 2008; Solomon et al. 2005) have also reported associations between combat, trauma, social support, and loneliness in a number of studies of Israeli veterans (combat and noncombat), as well as those of former prisoners of war. Some of their key findings include evidence that combat stress is associated with higher levels of loneliness and that loneliness may mediate a relationship between PTSD symptoms and marital discord (Itzhaky et al. 2017; Solomon and Dekel 2008). They also found that front-line treatment of combat stress might be effective in terms of reduced PTSD symptoms and loneliness up to 20 years later (Solomon et al. 2005).

Much of the research on PTSD symptoms and loneliness has focused on combat veterans. However, there is also an important relationship between interpersonal traumas, such as childhood sexual abuse, and loneliness. Research has pointed to a connection between childhood abuse, later loneliness, and mental health concerns, including PTSD (Shevlin et al. 2015). Such findings are also relevant to a PTSD syndrome first suggested in 1992 by Herman (1992) as "complex PTSD." Complex PTSD is not recognized in DSM-5-TR (American Psychiatric Association 2022) but is in the ICD-11 (World Health Organization 2019). In addition to the standard core of intrusion/recurrence, avoidance, and arousal symptoms, complex PTSD involves difficulties with affect regulation, self-concept, and interpersonal relations. All three of the additional defining symptom clusters have obvious relevance to the experience of loneliness. Notably, risk factors for complex PTSD include a history of childhood sexual abuse, physical abuse, neglect, and other early life or persistent inescapable traumas, largely those of an interpersonal nature. Dagan and Yager (2019) recently proposed that loneliness may have a key role in the development and maintenance of complex PTSD. Simon et al. (2019) found that participants with complex PTSD reported lower levels of perceived social support, but their study did not permit evaluation of the Dagan and Yager model.

If, as seems likely, loneliness and PTSD symptoms engage through reciprocal pathways, then treating loneliness in persons who have experienced a traumatic event may help prevent or reduce PTSD symptoms. As part of standard care, clinicians working with patients presenting with PTSD should generally evaluate and consider the array of traumatic events a person can experience, ranging from single-incident trauma to the types of long-term traumas thought to result in complex PTSD. Because there has been a dearth of research focused on loneliness in people with PTSD, the prevalence of loneliness and response to trauma-focused therapies such as prolonged exposure or cognitive processing therapy remain unknown. However, given the documented associations of loneliness with trauma and PTSD symptoms, it is advisable to directly ask patients about feelings of loneliness, their specific phenomenological experience of loneliness, and any associations between loneliness and the nature of their trauma, their specific symptoms or beliefs, and their responsiveness to treatment.

Assessment and Treatment

Assessment

Given the associations between mental health concerns and loneliness, we recommend that some explicit consideration of loneliness be incorporated into routine clinical care. If used judiciously, as a means of examining possible concerns rather than drawing conclusions or diagnoses or categorizing people as lonely or not lonely, examination of responses to individual items could potentially have utility as a starting point for discussing loneliness with a patient or client.

The most widely used instrument in loneliness research is the 20-item UCLA LS3 (Russell 1996). Scores on this scale range from 20 to 80. To avoid underreporting due to the stigma attached to loneliness, the scale does not actually use the word itself but, rather, describes experiences or feelings associated with being lonely. This may be helpful for identifying concerns among people who are hesitant to use the word itself. There are no cut points for categorizing level of loneliness on this scale that have been empirically validated against an appropriate criterion standard, so no cut scores exist that are appropriate for clinical use. Rather, clinicians might find responses to the individual items to be a useful adjunct to clinical interview in identifying areas for follow-up. For research purposes only, there is a category scheme first employed by Smith (1985) in which a score of 20–34=low loneliness, 25–49=moderate loneliness, 50–64=moderately high loneliness, and 65–80=high loneliness. Although Smith herself made a point of being clear that these divisions are arbitrary, they have been employed in studies of loneliness in people with cancer (Deckx et al. 2014; Perry 1990; Sevil et al. 2006; Smith 1985), and in at least one study of people with schizophrenia (Yildirim and Kavak Budak 2020), so they may be useful in facilitating communication and in facilitating comparison of different research samples.

Use of the full 20-item instrument may be impractical for routine screening of loneliness in some settings or contexts. Nonetheless, it remains the criterion standard against which any abbreviated versions are validated. Hughes et al. (2004) developed a 3-item version from the 1980 revised version of the UCLA LS3 for use in large population-based surveys. The 3-item version was endorsed for use in clinical settings in a report from the National Academies of Sciences, Engineering, and Medicine (2020). However, it employs exclusively negatively worded items and constricts the 20-item scale's four-point response range to three points, which results in poor discrimination of low versus moderate levels of loneliness. In their systematic review, Alsubheen et al. (2021) found only moderate-quality evidence for construct validity of the 3-item scale but high-quality evidence for validity of the 4-item (and 10-item) version. In situations in which the full 20-item scale is impractical, we favor use of the 4- or 10-item versions developed, validated, and recommended by the primary author of the 20-item version (Russell 1996, 2017). The 4- and 10-item versions retain the full four-point response range (facilitating conversion to the categories described earlier) and retain the balance of positively and negatively worded items. Our group found the 4-item scale useful in a large-scale survey of loneliness and aging (Nguyen et al. 2020).

Another widely used scale for research on loneliness is the De Jong Gierveld Loneliness Scale (De Jong and van Tilburg 1999). The original scale has 11 items, but there is also an abbreviated 6-item version. This scale was developed and validated in the Netherlands but has also been translated into English. The authors reported cut scores to define respondents as "not lonely," "moderately lonely," or "strongly lonely," but the study in which these cut scores were developed was conducted (and reported) in Dutch, so the generalizability to English-speaking persons is unknown (van Tilburg and De Jong Gierveld 1999). There is one other caveat regarding the subscales of this instrument. The authors of the scale found a two-factor solution for the scale items. These factors are sometimes described as subscales of social versus emotional loneliness. However, as the authors noted, the items on the "social loneliness" factor are all positively worded (e.g., "There is always someone I can talk to about my day-to-day problems"), whereas those on the "emotional loneliness" subscale are all negatively worded (e.g., "I miss having a really close friend"). In short, the two factors may reflect method variance rather than differences in the underlying subconstruct of loneliness type. These caveats aside, as with the UCLA LS3, examination of responses to these items may provide useful suggestions for points to follow up on during the clinical interview.

No structured or semistructured interviews presently have been developed or validated for clinical assessment of patient/client loneliness. In the absence of such tools, we recommend that mental health clinicians incorporate appropriate probes for and follow-up questions about loneliness as part of their standard intake interview process. Some aspects of social functioning are already commonly evaluated in the clinical intake process, such as marital status, relationships with family, and religious affiliations. It is also important to ask patients about their social support networks, such as close friends, people they see or with whom they talk on a regular basis (both at work and in their home lives), people (if any) with whom they feel emotionally close, and people to whom they turn when they need assistance or emotional or instrumental support. Open-ended questions about loneliness can be readily incorporated as part of this overall social-support evaluation. One way is to simply ask, "When is the last time you've felt lonely?" or "What does loneliness look/feel like to you?" followed by questions to encourage the person to describe the experience(s) and how their presenting concerns may affect or be affected by their relationships and feelings of loneliness.

If loneliness seems to be an important theme, it can be helpful to follow up with questions to identify any triggers for such feelings and the nature of the missing but desired aspects of their social relationships. Loneliness may also present in different types, for example, as part of a grief process or as anxiety about desired new relationships. Some distinguish between emotional and social loneliness—that is, yearning for intimate relationships or feeling distressed about one's broader network of close friends and connection to a broader community. All of these variations in theme and feelings can intersect with primary mental health concerns and thus should be considered over the course of treatment.

As stated earlier, some patients may not use or be comfortable with the use of the term *loneliness* because it carries some degree of stigma for them. With such individuals, it may be more helpful to evaluate feelings associated with loneliness, such as those of detachment, exclusion, or unpleasant isolation, rather than using the word *loneliness*. It is also important not to conflate loneliness with voluntary solitude. Solitude is not in itself a negative experience if it is genuinely desired by the person. This too is something patients can describe if asked.

Treatment

The purpose of assessing loneliness in the context of mental health care is to determine if the patient is experiencing a clinically relevant level of loneliness, the nature of that loneliness, and its intersection with their primary mental health concerns. Such assessment may also reveal the potential need for and points of intervention. There is a burgeoning body of research on loneliness-focused interventions (see Chapter 8, "Interventions for Loneliness in Younger People"; Chapter 9, "Interventions for Loneliness in Older Adults"; and Chapter 10, "Community-Based Interventions for Loneliness"). However, most of these interventions and intervention studies have focused on loneliness among older adults and the general population rather than in the context of mental health disorders. There have been more recent calls in the literature for a specific research agenda to develop, validate, and deploy loneliness-focused interventions in the context of mental health concerns (Jeste et al. 2020).

Although there are gaps in our current understanding of interventions for loneliness, loneliness concerns can still be addressed within the context of psychotherapeutic care. Depending on the specific needs and strengths of the individual patient, some points of intervention include objective social isolation, social skills or social cognitive skills, other cognitive distortions, and distorted beliefs about oneself or the meaning of solitude. The intersection of loneliness with primary symptoms, such as depressive thought patterns, mania/hypomania, social anxiety, positive and negative symptoms of psychoses, and trauma, is a potentially relevant point of biological and psychotherapeutic intervention. Given the high rates of medical comorbidity with mental health disorders, the association of loneliness with any medical concern, such as chronic pain, substance use, and acute or chronic medical conditions, should also be considered.

Mental health disorders may adversely impact social functioning and lead to higher levels of social isolation, loneliness, or both. It is important to assess each component because they may have independent or related implications. Improving social engagement may be helpful to reduce loneliness in those individuals for whom objective isolation is the critical factor. For those who prefer solitude, however, efforts to increase social engagement can have adverse effects on well-being unless the factors underlying such a preference are first explored. For others, it may be necessary to address maladaptive beliefs and distorted social perceptions sustaining loneliness. As noted by Cacioppo and Hawkley (2005):

> people may *become* lonely due to an unfortunate event but *remain* lonely because of the manner in which they and others think about each other—their social cognition—their social expectations and aspirations, the way they perceive others, and the manner in which they process, remember, appraise, and act on social information. (p. 98; italics in original)

The reaction of others may be influenced by stigma and fear about loneliness and about mental illness, but lonely people may also have a self-stigma and dysfunctional social cognitions that may be addressed through cognitive or cognitive-behavioral therapies.

The following case vignettes provide two examples of how considerations of loneliness can be relevant to the care of individuals with mental health concerns.

Nicholas

Nicholas was a 25-year-old white male who sought psychotherapy treatment at the request of his mother because of the sudden loss of his father. He was a second-year law student in a major metropolitan city and lived alone, was not in a romantic relationship, and his family lived across the country in a different state. He explained that he was at the top of his class at a very prestigious law school, had an internship with "one of the best criminal defense attorneys" in his city, and was president of numerous clubs at his law school. He maintained that despite his father's passing, he was still actively involved in all of these roles because "they are a good distraction." He reported feeling "normal" his whole life and has never believed he needed therapy.

During the initial psychotherapy session, Nicholas reported a loss of appetite, trouble falling asleep, and loss of pleasure for leisure activities since his father's passing. He also reported recent feelings of intense anger and anger outbursts followed by periods of social withdrawal and feelings of emptiness. Nicholas explained that these symptoms of anger had occurred more frequently since his father passed away. They usually increased when he thought about his father's sudden passing because he "wasn't able to say goodbye" and because being the executor of his father's will has caused added stress. Immediately after his father's passing, Nicholas threw his phone over a balcony and deleted all of his social media because he "wanted to be left alone" and "didn't want to deal" with people offering their sympathies. He expressed increased feelings of isolation and loneliness since his father's passing but would "rather not tell his friends how [he's] feeling because [he] doesn't want to burden them." Nicholas reported a very robust social life but believed his friends had been distancing themselves from him lately due to the increased frequency of his anger outbursts. He became embarrassed by his anger when it occurred in front of his friends, which led him to further withdraw. Because he lived away from his family, he predominantly relied on his friends for social support. He reduced contact with his mother and sister because they always wanted to talk about the passing of his father, and he "can't deal with their emotions." He denied a history of suicide attempts or ideation and denied a history of nonsuicidal self-injury.

The early focus of psychotherapy was to identify and better understand how Nicholas's grief and depressive symptoms from his father's sudden loss were interrelated with his feelings of loneliness and social withdrawal. During the initial visit, the clinician administered the (20-item) UCLA LS3, on which Nicholas endorsed many of the items indicative of multiple feelings relevant to loneliness. The clinician followed up with Nicholas during the intake interview to ask him about feelings of loss and loneliness, and Nicholas decided that these were among the concerns he wanted to address in his treatment The clinician worked with Nicholas to develop a treatment plan that included cognitive therapy to identify maladaptive thoughts, including feelings of guilt, and to teach him a mindful self-compassion meditation to promote self-acceptance. After several psychotherapy sessions, Nicholas reported that he was having greater feelings of connection with his friends and that he was using a teleconferencing platform to better connect with his family members. Nicholas was more accepting of his father's sudden death and recognized that he was not at fault for what had happened. He was able to understand his anger as a part of his bereavement. The clinician taught Nicholas skills to acknowledge and manage his feelings of anger before they became an unmanageable outburst. Nicholas began trying different hobbies, such as hiking, which led him to find pleasure again in activities he previously enjoyed, which also broadened his social network. As Nicholas began to make progress on working on his grief, he was more able to effectively communicate his feelings without getting dysregulated, leading to repaired relationships with his friends and family.

Lila

Lila was a 36-year-old female military veteran. She had been diagnosed with PTSD after returning from Afghanistan. She was married to an officer in the army and had no children. She and her husband had recently moved to a new town, where she was a substitute teacher at her local high school. She sought psychotherapy from a clinical psychologist, "not because of her combat history" but for feelings of extreme social isolation. In her initial psychotherapy visit, Lila described that throughout her youth she had experienced emotional and physical abuse from her mother, who had a substance abuse problem and was an "absent parent." Lila explained that she had joined the military to escape her family situation. While she was in basic training, Lila reported multiple incidences of sexual harassment by her male colleagues. During this time, she felt increasingly socially isolated from her colleagues due to this harassment. She felt unable to report it to her superiors because she did not want to create more problems for herself. During her first active-duty tour in Afghanistan, she witnessed things "no person is equipped to see." She also completed a second tour of Afghanistan because she thought no one else would understand what she had gone through the first time and felt that she was "doing something fulfilling and worthwhile by serving [her] country." Shortly after finishing her second tour, she met her husband through a mutual army friend. She stated that her husband was away frequently and for long periods of time because of his job. She endorsed a past history of suicide ideation but denied current suicidality. She had never engaged in self-injurious behavior. She stated that her most prolonged periods of suicide ideation were during basic training and after her second tour in Afghanistan, when she sought treatment for PTSD. She maintained that her PTSD had been successfully treated with twice-weekly psychotherapy and a selective serotonin reuptake inhibitor. Lila maintained that she no longer experienced PTSD and considered herself "high functioning" because of her success at her job and her marriage.

During her initial psychotherapy visit, Lila reported that her mother had returned to her life after becoming sober, seeking to have a relationship with her. Lila explained that her mother's side of the family was extremely receptive to her mother's sobriety and that she had felt "pressured" to start a relationship with her, despite the family's knowledge of their turbulent relationship. Lila had ceased contact with her family as a result and felt "abandoned" by them for "choosing her over me" and being "quick to forgive her." She was "at a loss" because her husband was away and difficult to contact. She lived in a new town where she did not have friends. She explained that she was "used to dealing with things alone," but this time she needed help.

The early focus of psychotherapy was to identify how Lila's extensive trauma history with her family and her time in the military contributed to her feelings of loneliness and social isolation, and how social isolation and loneliness were independent components of her trauma history. During the initial visit, the clinician administered the De Jong Gierveld Loneliness Scale, on which Lila endorsed items consistent with social and emotional loneliness; these concerns were confirmed on further discussion during the intake interview. The psychologist worked with Lila to develop a treatment plan that included cognitive-behavioral therapy to catch, check, and change her maladaptive thought patterns and responses. It also included behavioral activation exercises to help Lila identify active steps for connecting with other women veterans who had experienced interpersonal trauma. After several psychotherapy sessions, Lila decided that she was ready to consider reestablishing her relationship with her mother and her family. She set a goal to have her mother visit her and spend time with her by the end of the year so that they could explore a new relationship together. She also decided to join local community organizations for veterans and began taking dance classes, which helped expand her social network. As Lila became more active in her community and worked through her familial and military trauma history, she became more engaged socially and more motivated to repair her relationship with her mother.

Summary

Loneliness is a common human experience and an importantly adaptive one as a motivator for social connection. However, when acute loneliness becomes chronic and persistent, it can quickly snowball, triggering a cascade of problems such as dysfunctional and distorted social cognitions or sustained heightened arousal that may lead to adverse health outcomes. Many of the most common mental health disorders are associated with elevated risk for chronic loneliness and social isolation. The adverse health outcomes associated with disorders such as schizophrenia and PTSD overlap with those associated with loneliness. Further research to clarify the temporal associations between these relationships and distinct points of intervention are imperative. The key for clinicians in mental health settings is to ask patients about loneliness and social connection and to recognize problems or concerns that they are experiencing because of loneliness and low social support.

There is an important need for systematic research to understand the nature of loneliness in the context of mental health disorders. For example, most of the existing research on loneliness among people living with mental health conditions has focused on scores from quantitative loneliness rating scales, but there is a clear and pressing need to complement such data with qualitative research for a more in-depth understanding of the triggers for and internal phenomenological experience of loneliness (McKenna-Plumley et al. 2020; Morlett Paredes et al. 2020). It is in this aspect that the nuances of loneliness may vary most across different categories of mental health disorders and between individuals within those categories. There also remain basic unanswered questions, such as the frequency of problematic loneliness in disorders such as bipolar disorder and PTSD. More nuanced research is needed on preferences for solitude in the context of depression, anxiety, schizophrenia, and PTSD because these stated preferences can sometimes represent a form of avoidance of stress and negative feelings resulting from attempts at connection—that is, a form of "learned helplessness." In these individuals there may be a desire for connection but also feelings of fear or hopelessness about such connection. For other individuals, or in the same individuals at other times, there may be positive aspects of voluntary solitude that should be respected, whereas other individuals may find it difficult to tolerate solitude due to fears and distorted thoughts about what it "means" to be alone. These are all points of potential intervention.

Our focus in this chapter has been on the intersection of loneliness with primary mental health disorders. However, it is also important to consider that chronic physical health concerns can add to the complex relationship of loneliness and mental well-being. For example, problems with increased loneliness have been identified in people with chronic pain, cancer, traumatic brain injury, spinal cord injury, psoriasis, and irritable bowel syndrome. There are multiple potential routes by which various physical conditions might affect social isolation and loneliness, including decreases in mobility and physical function, as well as self-perceived stigma. The potential intersection and interaction of primary mental health concerns, loneliness, and social isolation, together with the social impact of chronic medical concerns, can feel overwhelmingly complex. However, keeping each of these possibilities in mind while working in partnership with each individual patient can help the clinician identify an order of priorities. The bottom line is to ask each patient about feelings of loneliness and if and how the patient's mental and physical health, lived experience, and self-identified core dimensions of self-identity may interact and be relevant to an overall treatment plan.

KEY POINTS

- Prevalence rates of loneliness among people with mental health disorders are higher than those in the general public.

- The nuances of how loneliness is initiated, maintained, and experienced may vary across different mental health disorders and will naturally differ among individuals within each category.

- There are important gaps in the empirical literature on loneliness in this population, but existing evidence is sufficient to support universal screening for the potential presence of loneliness and social isolation in mental health care settings.

- Inclusion of brief screening instruments for loneliness and social isolation and consideration of these factors in clinical interviews and clinician–patient discussions during the course of treatment should be routine components of comprehensive mental health care.

Suggested Readings

Eglit GML, Palmer BW, Martin AS, et al: Loneliness in schizophrenia: construct clarification, measurement, and clinical relevance. PLoS One 13(3):e0194021, 2018 29566046

Erzen E, Çikrikci Ö: The effect of loneliness on depression: a meta-analysis. Int J Soc Psychiatry 64(5):427–435, 2018 29792097

Gentry M, Palmer BW: The "timbre" of loneliness in late life. Int Psychogeriatr 33(12):1233–1236, 2021

Lim MH, Penn DL, Thomas N, Gleeson JFM: Is loneliness a feasible treatment target in psychosis? Soc Psychiatry Psychiatr Epidemiol 55(7):901–906, 2020 31127348

Straus E, Norman SB, Tripp JC, et al: Behavioral epidemic of loneliness in older U.S. military veterans: results from the 2019–2020 National Health and Resilience in Veterans Study. Am J Geriatr Psychiatry 30(3):297–310, 2022 34417085

References

Abdellaoui A, Nivard MG, Hottenga JJ, et al: Predicting loneliness with polygenic scores of social, psychological and psychiatric traits. Genes Brain Behav 17(6):e12472, 2018 29573219

Adams KB, Sanders S, Auth EA: Loneliness and depression in independent living retirement communities: risk and resilience factors. Aging Ment Health 8(6):475–485, 2004 15724829

Alsubheen SA, Oliveira A, Habash R, et al: Systematic review of psychometric properties and cross-cultural adaptation of the University of California and Los Angeles loneliness scale in adults. Curr Psychol 2021 34785877 Epub ahead of print

American Psychiatric Association: Diagnostic and Statistical Manual of Mental Disorders, 5th Edition, Text Revision. Washington, DC, American Psychiatric Association, 2022

Badcock JC, Shah S, Mackinnon A, et al: Loneliness in psychotic disorders and its association with cognitive function and symptom profile. Schizophr Res 169(1–3):268–273, 2015 26527247

Badcock JC, Di Prinzio P, Waterreus A, et al: Loneliness and its association with health service utilization in people with a psychotic disorder. Schizophr Res 223:105–111, 2020 32518000

Beebe LH: What community living problems do persons with schizophrenia report during periods of stability? Perspect Psychiatr Care 46(1):48–55, 2010 20051078

Cacioppo JT, Hawkley LC: People thinking about people: the vicious cycle of being a social outcast in one's own mind, in The Social Outcast: Ostracism, Social Exclusion, Rejection, and Bullying. Edited by Williams KD, Forgas JP, von Hippel W. New York, Psychology Press, 2005, pp 91–108

Cacioppo JT, Patrick W: Loneliness: Human Nature and the Need for Social Connection. New York, W.W. Norton and Co, 2008

Cacioppo JT, Hawkley LC, Ernst JM, et al: Loneliness within a nomological net: an evolutionary perspective. J Res Pers 40(6):1054–1085, 2006

Cacioppo S, Grippo AJ, London S, et al: Loneliness: clinical import and interventions. Perspect Psychol Sci 10(2):238–249, 2015 25866548

Chau AKC, Zhu C, So SH: Loneliness and the psychosis continuum: a meta-analysis on positive psychotic experiences and a meta-analysis on negative psychotic experiences. Int Rev Psychiatry 31(5-6):471–490, 2019 31331209

Cornwell EY, Waite LJ: Measuring social isolation among older adults using multiple indicators from the NSHAP study. J Gerontol B Psychol Sci Soc Sci 64(suppl 1):i38–i46, 2009 19508982

Dagan Y, Yager J: Addressing loneliness in complex PTSD. J Nerv Ment Dis 207(6):433–439, 2019 31045977

Davidson L, Stayner D: Loss, loneliness, and the desire for love: perspectives on the social lives of people with schizophrenia. Psychiatr Rehabil J 20(3):3–12, 1997

De Jong J, van Tilburg T: Manual of the Loneliness Scale. Amsterdam, Vrije Universiteit Department of Social Research Methodology, 1999

de Siqueira Rotenberg L, Beraldi GH, Okawa Belizario G, Lafer B: Impaired social cognition in bipolar disorder: a meta-analysis of theory of mind in euthymic patients. Aust N Z J Psychiatry 54(8):783–796, 2020 32447967

Deckx L, van den Akker M, Buntinx F: Risk factors for loneliness in patients with cancer: a systematic literature review and meta-analysis. Eur J Oncol Nurs 18(5):466–477, 2014 24993076

Domènech-Abella J, Mundó J, Haro JM, Rubio-Valera M: Anxiety, depression, loneliness and social network in the elderly: longitudinal associations from The Irish Longitudinal Study on Ageing (TILDA). J Affect Disord 246:82–88, 2019 30578950

Eglit GML, Palmer BW, Martin AS, et al: Loneliness in schizophrenia: construct clarification, measurement, and clinical relevance. PloS One 13(3):e0194021, 2018 29566046

Erzen E, Çikrikci Ö: The effect of loneliness on depression: a meta-analysis. Int J Soc Psychiatry 64(5):427–435, 2018 29792097

Fortuna KL, Ferron J, Pratt SI, et al. Unmet needs of people with serious mental illness: perspectives from certified peer specialists. Psychiatr Q 90(3):579–586, 2019 31154551

Fox R, Power J, Coogan A, et al: Posttraumatic stress disorder and loneliness are associated over time: a longitudinal study on PTSD symptoms and loneliness, among older adults. Psychiatry Res 299:113846, 2021 33706195

Gard DE, Kring AM, Gard MG, et al: Anhedonia in schizophrenia: distinctions between anticipatory and consummatory pleasure. Schizophr Res 93(1–3):253–260, 2007 17490858

Goossens L, van Roekel E, Verhagen M, et al: The genetics of loneliness: linking evolutionary theory to genome-wide genetics, epigenetics, and social science. Perspect Psychol Sci 10(2):213–226, 2015 25910391

Granek L, Danan D, Bersudsky Y, Osher Y: Living with bipolar disorder: the impact on patients, spouses, and their marital relationship. Bipolar Disord 18(2):192–199, 2016 26890335

Green MF, Horan WP, Lee J, et al: Social disconnection in schizophrenia and the general community. Schizophr Bull 44(2):242–249, 2018 28637195

Grover S, Nehra R, Thakur A: Bipolar affective disorder and its impact on various aspects of marital relationship. Ind Psychiatry J 26(2):114–120, 2017 30089956

Hawkley LC, Masi CM, Berry JD, Cacioppo JT: Loneliness is a unique predictor of age-related differences in systolic blood pressure. Psychol Aging 21(1):152–164, 2006 16594800

Herman JL: Complex PTSD: a syndrome in survivors of prolonged and repeated trauma. J Trauma Stress 5(3):377–391, 1992

Holt-Lunstad J: The major health implications of social connection. Curr Dir Psychol Sci 30(3):251–259, 2021

Holwerda TJ, Deeg DJH, Beekman ATF, et al: Feelings of loneliness, but not social isolation, predict dementia onset: results from the Amsterdam Study of the Elderly (AMSTEL). J Neurol Neurosurg Psychiatry 85(2):135–142, 2014

Holwerda TJ, van Tilburg TG, Deeg DJH, et al: Impact of loneliness and depression on mortality: results from the Longitudinal Ageing Study Amsterdam. Br J Psychiatry 209(2):127–134, 2016 27103680

Hughes ME, Waite LJ, Hawkley LC, Cacioppo JT: A short scale for measuring loneliness in large surveys: results from two population-based studies. Res Aging 26(6):655–672, 2004 18504506

Itzhaky L, Stein JY, Levin Y, Solomon Z: Posttraumatic stress symptoms and marital adjustment among Israeli combat veterans: the role of loneliness and attachment. Psychol Trauma 9(6):655–662, 2017 28206786

Jeste DV, Lee EE, Cacioppo S: Battling the modern behavioral epidemic of loneliness: suggestions for research and interventions. JAMA Psychiatry 77(6):553–554, 2020 32129811

Kamarsu S, Kauffman C, Palmer BW, Depp CA: Ecological momentary assessment of social activity in bipolar disorder. J Behav Cogn Ther 30(1):41–48, 2020

Kuwert P, Knaevelsrud C, Pietrzak RH: Loneliness among older veterans in the United States: results from the National Health and Resilience in Veterans Study. Am J Geriatr Psychiatry 22(6):564–569, 2014 23806682

Lee SL, Pearce E, Ajnakina O, et al: The association between loneliness and depressive symptoms among adults aged 50 years and older: a 12-year population-based cohort study. Lancet Psychiatry 8(1):48–57, 2021 33181096

Lim MH, Rodebaugh TL, Zyphur MJ, Gleeson JF: Loneliness over time: the crucial role of social anxiety. J Abnorm Psychol 125(5):620–630, 2016 27124713

Lim MH, Gleeson JF, Rodebaugh TL, et al: A pilot digital intervention targeting loneliness in young people with psychosis. Soc Psychiatry Psychiatr Epidemiol 55(7):877–889, 2020a 30874828

Lim MH, Penn DL, Thomas N, Gleeson JF. Is loneliness a feasible treatment target in psychosis? Soc Psychiatry Psychiatr Epidemiol 55(7):901–906, 2020b 31127348

McKenna-Plumley PE, Groarke JM, Turner RN, Yang K: Experiences of loneliness: a study protocol for a systematic review and thematic synthesis of qualitative literature. Syst Rev 9(1):284, 2020 33280605

Michalska da Rocha B, Rhodes S, Vasilopoulou E, Hutton P: Loneliness in psychosis: a meta-analytical review. Schizophr Bull 44(1):114–125, 2018 28369646

Morgan VA, Waterreus A, Carr V, et al: Responding to challenges for people with psychotic illness: updated evidence from the Survey of High Impact Psychosis. Aust N Z J Psychiatry 51(2):124–140, 2017 27913580

Morlett Paredes A, Lee EE, Chik L, et al: Qualitative study of loneliness in a senior housing community: the importance of wisdom and other coping strategies. Aging Ment Health 25(3):559–566, 2020 31918561

National Academies of Sciences, Engineering, and Medicine: Social Isolation and Loneliness in Older Adults: Opportunities for the Health Care System. Washington, DC, The National Academies Press, 2020

Nguyen TT, Lee EE, Daly RE, et al: Predictors of loneliness by age decade: study of psychological and environmental factors in 2,843 community-dwelling Americans aged 20–69 years. J Clin Psychiatry 81(6):20m13378, 2020 33176072

Owen R, Gooding P, Dempsey R, Jones S: The reciprocal relationship between bipolar disorder and social interaction: a qualitative investigation. Clin Psychol Psychother 24(4):911–918, 2017 27862615

Perry GR: Loneliness and coping among tertiary-level adult cancer patients in the home. Cancer Nurs 13(5):293–302, 1990 2245416

Rico-Uribe LA, Caballero FF, Martin-Maria N, et al: Association of loneliness with all-cause mortality: a meta-analysis. PLoS One 13(1):e0190033, 2018 29300743

Roe D, Mashiach-Eizenberg M, Lysaker PH: The relation between objective and subjective domains of recovery among persons with schizophrenia-related disorders. Schizophr Res 131(1–3):133–138, 2011 21669512

Rook KS: Interventions for loneliness: a review and analysis, in Preventing the Harmful Consequences of Severe and Persistent Loneliness. Edited by Peplau LA, Goldston SE. Rockville, MD, U.S. Dept. of Health and Human Services, Public Health Service, Alcohol, Drug Abuse, and Mental Health Administration, National Institute of Mental Health, 1984, pp 47–94

Russell DW: UCLA Loneliness Scale (Version 3): reliability, validity, and factor structure. J Pers Assess 66(1):20–40, 1996 8576833

Russell DW: Normative data for the UCLA Loneliness Scale. Ames, IA, Department of Human Development and Family Studies, Iowa State University, 2017

Russell DW, Peplau LA, Cutrona CE: The revised UCLA Loneliness Scale: concurrent and discriminant validity evidence. J Pers Soc Psychol 39(3):472–480, 1980 7431205

Sevil U, Ertem G, Kavlak O, Coban A: The loneliness level of patients with gynecological cancer. Int J Gynecol Cancer 16 (suppl 1):472–477, 2006 16515647

Shao R, Liu HL, Huang CM, et al: Loneliness and depression dissociated on parietal-centered networks in cognitive and resting states. Psychol Med 50(16):2691–2701, 2020 31615593

Shevlin M, McElroy E, Murphy J: Loneliness mediates the relationship between childhood trauma and adult psychopathology: evidence from the adult psychiatric morbidity survey. Soc Psychiatry Psychiatr Epidemiol 50(4):591–601, 2015 25208908

Shumway M, Unick GJ, McConnell WA, et al: Measuring community preferences for public mental health services: pilot test of a mail survey method. Community Ment Health J 40(4):281–295, 2004 15453082

Simon N, Roberts NP, Lewis CE, et al: Associations between perceived social support, posttraumatic stress disorder (PTSD) and complex PTSD (CPTSD): implications for treatment. Eur J Psychotraumatol 10(1):1573129, 2019 30788064

Smith S: Measurement of Loneliness Among Clients Representing Four Stages of Cancer: An Exploratory Study. Wright-Patterson AFB, OH, Air Force Institute of Technology, 1985

Solomon Z, Dekel R: The contribution of loneliness and posttraumatic stress disorder to marital adjustment following war captivity: a longitudinal study. Fam Process 47(2):261–275, 2008 18605125

Solomon Z, Shklar R, Mikulincer M: Frontline treatment of combat stress reaction: a 20-year longitudinal evaluation study. Am J Psychiatry 162(12):2309–2314, 2005 16330595

Spithoven AWM, Cacioppo S, Goossens L, Cacioppo JT: Genetic contributions to loneliness and their relevance to the evolutionary theory of loneliness. Perspect Psychol Sci 14(3):376–396, 2019 30844327

Stain HJ, Galletly CA, Clark S, et al: Understanding the social costs of psychosis: the experience of adults affected by psychosis identified within the second Australian National Survey of Psychosis. Aust N Z J Psychiatry 46(9):879–889, 2012 22645395

Stek ML, Vinkers DJ, Gussekloo J, et al: Is depression in old age fatal only when people feel lonely? Am J Psychiatry 162(1):178–180, 2005 15625218

van der Velden PG, Pijnappel B, van der Meulen E: Correction to: potentially traumatic events have negative and positive effects on loneliness, depending on PTSD-symptom levels: evidence from a population-based prospective comparative study. Soc Psychiatry Psychiatr Epidemiol 53(5):541–543, 2018 29520476

van Tilburg TG, De Jong Gierveld J: [Reference standards for the loneliness scale]. Tijdschr Gerontol Geriatr 30(4):158–163, 1999 10486620

Wang J, Lloyd-Evans B, Marston L, et al: Epidemiology of loneliness in a cohort of UK mental health community crisis service users. Soc Psychiatry Psychiatr Epidemiol 55(7):811–822, 2019 31222412

Warren CD, Fowler K, Speed D, Walsh A: The influence of social support on psychological distress in Canadian adults with bipolar disorder. Soc Psychiatry Psychiatr Epidemiol 53(8):815–821, 2018 29737385

Weeks DG, Michela JL, Peplau LA, Bragg ME: Relation between loneliness and depression: a structural equation analysis. J Pers Soc Psychol 39(6):1238–1244, 1980 7205551

World Health Organization: International Statistical Classification of Diseases and Related Health Problems, 11th Edition. Geneva, World Health Organization, 2019

Yildirim T, Kavak Budak F: The relationship between internalized stigma and loneliness in patients with schizophrenia. Perspect Psychiatr Care 56(1):168–174, 2020 31093994

Loneliness in Marginalized Communities

Lize Tibiriçá, Psy.D.
Dylan J. Jester, Ph.D., M.P.H.
Barton W. Palmer, Ph.D.
Dilip V. Jeste, M.D.

SOME HISTORIANS suggest that the contemporary concept of (and word for) loneliness in Western societies emerged with the rise of secularism and changes in social relationships secondary to industrialization (Alberti 2019). However, the capacity to experience some form of distress signal in response to perceived social isolation or disconnection was likely favored by natural selection because it serves as a social motivating signal for behaviors that increase the probability of connection, survival, and reproduction (Cacioppo and Cacioppo 2018). The concept of loneliness is thus a key example of an experience that is partially driven by biology but also highly influenced by environment, experience, and culture.

Concern about what seems to be a contemporary "pandemic" of loneliness and social isolation, along with associated suicidality and opioid abuse, is notably not restricted to any one part of the globe (Jeste et al. 2020). Studies of loneliness are being conducted in many countries and cultures. In addition to questions about how culture may affect the prevalence of persistent loneliness, there are also key questions about how culture may affect the internal phenomenological experience of loneliness. It is plausible that identification with a collectivist rather than an individualist culture could be either a protective or a risk factor for loneliness, depending on one's feeling of belongingness and connection within the community (Barreto et al. 2021). There indeed are data showing a protective effect of group identification (e.g., degree of ethnic identity) that may result in a sense of community stronger than that typical in the majority U.S. culture (Salway et al. 2020). On the other hand, cultural expectations of connection can impact loneliness if people believe that they are not meeting the expectations of their culture. Consideration of existing quantitative and qualitative data may be helpful in validly disentangling the multitude of potential interacting factors.

Although much of the research on loneliness from North America has focused on samples that predominantly comprise cisgender heterosexual non-Latinx white adults, there are strong reasons to suspect that experiences of marginalization, bigotry, and discrimination may also impact subjective and objective aspects of social isolation (Salway et al. 2020). As noted elsewhere in this volume, chronic loneliness not only is an adverse experience that negatively affects emotional well-being but also has substantial deleterious biological effects that manifest in terms of medical comorbidity and early mortality. Yet complex but critical questions arise when trying to generalize findings from loneliness research on relatively homogeneous nonmarginalized persons to those in various marginalized groups.

In this chapter we present an overview, grounded in relevant empirical literature, of the interaction of culture and discrimination/marginalization on the prevalence and experience of loneliness, risk and protective factors, and downstream impact on health, well-being, and mortality (Holt-Lunstad et al. 2015). In providing this overview we do not imply monolithic within-group experiences, attitudes, or beliefs. Rather, our goal is to offer clinicians and other readers a list of factors and dimensions that warrant consideration when working with persons from diverse backgrounds. There is obviously a multitude of dimensions in which diversity and marginalization may exist, such as race, sex, religion/faith, nationality, health or physical function (e.g., persons with physical disabilities), and the like. For the present chapter, our focus is on communities that are marginalized because of their cultural background, socioeconomic status, ethnicity/race, gender identity, sexual orientation, and migration status. We recognize that these are not orthogonal categories but, rather, tend to intersect with one another and with other factors in a particular person. We consider both what is known about these factors from the existing empirical literature and gaps in current knowledge/directions for research. We summarize findings from studies in the Hispanic/Latinx, Black, immigrant, and LGBTQ+ communities and then provide brief recommendations for future work.

Hispanic/Latinx Community

In 2015, approximately two-thirds of Hispanic/Latinx individuals in the United States were U.S.-born (Noe-Bustamante and Flores 2019). Some studies have reported that Hispanic/Latinx adults experience higher levels of loneliness than Black and white adults (Hawkley et al. 2008), whereas other studies have found no significant difference in loneliness by race or ethnicity (Compernolle et al. 2021; Tomaka et al. 2006). It has been suggested that household income and education explain, in part, the association between loneliness and race/ethnicity (Hawkley et al. 2008). Racial and ethnic categories reflect a set of experiences and stress exposures within social and physical environments. Financial difficulties are among the many stressors that result from both minority status and the migration experience (Caplan 2007; Hurtado-de-Mendoza et al. 2014). Structural sources of stress, such as financial strain, can influence health both by acting as a source of stress and by truncating the opportunities or protective resources individuals have to cope with stressors such as loneliness. Other stressors might include language barriers and changes in or loss of interpersonal relationships and social support.

Hispanic/Latinx adults report experiences of discrimination, and new or recent immigrants may also experience an added layer of culture shock. The Latinx community is described as collectivist and family oriented (Sue and Sue 2016), valuing *familialismo*, which reflects the importance of extended families/relatives for several aspects of life and community, including support and guidance, childcare, and family-related responsibilities (Dominguez-Fuentes and Hombrados-Mendieta 2012). The U.S. values of individualism and autonomy may challenge those collectivist values, and Hispanic/Latinx immigrants might not be able to live in accordance with their values because they lack family members nearby and experience changes in their nuclear family (e.g., when one parent moves with the child and the other parent remains in the country of origin).

According to Perreira et al. (2006), Hispanic/Latinx immigrant parents can experience a loss of support system and grief. Childcare responsibilities also might change as a result of migration (Parsai et al. 2006; Villar 2010). In addition to loneliness, parents might experience fear, sadness, and burnout (Ansion and Merali 2018). However, positive changes might also result from the immigration experience. In a small study of 10 Latinx parents who moved to Canada, parents reported an initial experience of negative emotions such as fear, worry, and sadness in addition to loneliness and burnout.

As a result of those experiences and the absence of extended family, however, parents sought new ways of parenting alongside their partners, which led to an increase in nuclear family cohesion. Another positive change these parents experienced related to the fact that fathers appeared to become more involved in childrearing (Ansion and Merali 2018).

Physical Health and Loneliness

Hispanic/Latinx adults experiencing loneliness might be at a greater risk for cardiovascular disease (e.g., hypertension, heart disease, stroke) (Tomaka et al. 2006) and metabolic dysregulation (e.g., metabolic burden, increased BMI, glycated hemoglobin/HbA1c) (Shiovitz-Ezra and Parag 2019). The relationship between loneliness and cardiovascular disease was reported in another study with only Latinx individuals (Foti et al. 2020). In this study, lonely adults were at risk of developing cardiovascular diseases (OR 1.10, 95% CI 1.01–1.20, $P<0.05$) and diabetes mellitus (OR 1.08, 95% CI 1.00–1.16, $P<0.05$). These associations remained significant after adjusting for depression, smoking status, demographics, and BMI. However, age, sex, marital status, and number of years in the United States did not moderate the associations.

Loneliness was also found to be positively associated with high systolic blood pressure in a study by Hawkley et al. (2010), and this association was independent of several variables, including sociodemographic variables, cardiovascular risk factors, medications, health conditions, and the effects of depressive symptoms, social support, perceived stress, and hostility. In this study, non-Black Latinx adults were 29% of the participants (the majority were of Mexican ethnicity, 72%). About 36% non-Hispanic white adults and 35% African American adults born between 1935 and 1952 and living in Cook County, Illinois, also participated in this study.

Hispanic/Latinx adults are more likely to live with others and to endorse family support (Tomaka et al. 2006), and those who are married and have someone to rely on or talk to report lower levels of loneliness (Gerst-Emerson et al. 2014). These could be protective factors in the development of certain medical conditions. Spirituality might also be a protective factor against health decline through lower levels of loneliness among Latinx individuals (Gallegos and Segrin 2019).

Mental Health, Interpersonal Factors, and Loneliness

Loneliness is also experienced by Hispanic/Latinx children. Surprisingly, middle school children experiencing high levels of loneliness also experienced high levels of well-being (Heredia et al. 2017). Peer and family support were two protective factors that moderated this association. There were also gender differences, with girls reporting more friends and boys reporting feeling less lonely.

As in other groups, loneliness is associated with depression in the Hispanic/Latinx community. Those with lower levels of loneliness experience lower levels of depression (Martinez et al. 2019). Furthermore, a study with Mexican American adults showed that individuals experiencing loneliness were at risk for experiencing changes in interpersonal relationships and cognitive functioning, perceiving their health as fair/poor, and an increase in depressive symptoms (Gerst-Emerson et al. 2014).

The presence of loneliness and negative life events can contribute to hopelessness and suicidal behaviors in the Hispanic/Latinx community. Investigators found that loneliness accounted for 24%–29% of variance in both outcomes, whereas negative life events accounted for about 3% of the variance in hopelessness only. Another study, focusing on Latinx college students, identified that ethnic identity and loneliness could predict suicidal behavior (Chang et al. 2017). These findings suggest that persons with a low sense of belonging to their own ethnic group and feeling lonely could be at a higher risk for suicide. Clinicians and other health care providers should evaluate loneliness and negative life events when assessing suicidality because these factors could contribute to the experience of hopelessness and suicidal behaviors.

Hispanic/Latinx adults with more support and lower levels of loneliness appear to be more resilient (Lee et al. 2020). Thus, having greater social support might help Hispanic/Latinx immigrants cope with the challenges they face and protect against social isolation and its negative consequences. Language barriers for Spanish-speaking people might also be a factor to consider in the risk of experiencing loneliness among Latinx communities. For instance, Hispanic/Latinx individuals who speak both English and Spanish fluently are more likely to report lower levels of loneliness. However, those who were less fluent in Spanish than English reported higher experience of loneliness.

Black/African American Community

Black adults compose 14% of the U.S. population, and more than half live in the South (Tamir 2021). In 2019, 35% of the U.S. Black population was under the age of 22, and 10% was under the age of 6. Among those identifying as Black-Latinx, an even greater share of the population was younger than 22 years (51%) and 6 years (18%), respectively (Tamir 2021). There have been some changes in mean education levels during recent decades. Black children and adolescents now have a greater likelihood of completing a college education than previous birth cohorts. Since 2000, the proportion of Black adults with at least an undergraduate degree increased from 15% in 2000 to 23% in 2019 (Tamir 2021). Although strides are being made by federal and state authorities to close educational achievement gaps, income inequality persists. In 2019, 29% of Black households in the United States made less than $25,000 annually, and 54% made less than $50,000, despite growing shares of adults achieving higher education (Tamir 2021).

It is well-known that Black adults in the United States are exposed to greater inequalities in education, environmental health, income, mental health, and physical health than white adults, and these inequalities culminate in a loss of upward mobility across successive generations (Chetty et al. 2020; Hamilton et al. 2015). Although this chapter focuses on loneliness and social disconnection among marginalized communities, it is important to understand that the discrimination and exploitation of Black adults (e.g., overt and covert discrimination, "redlining" districts to restrict economic mobility, urbanization without equitable access) have long-lasting effects that may ultimately contribute to continued disparities in mental health and loneliness today.

Loneliness is associated with poorer mental health, self-rated health, and quality of life among Black adults (Fisher et al. 2014; Wippold et al. 2021). However, the literature is mixed regarding whether Black adults are more likely to be lonely than white adults. In an urban sample from Minneapolis, Minnesota, Finlay and Kobayashi (2018) found that white adults were more than twice as likely to be lonely as Black adults (35% and 16%, respectively). Population-based studies have found that older Black adults were more lonely, more socially disconnected, had greater perceived isolation, and had smaller social networks than older white adults (Cornwell et al. 2008). These social networks tend to decrease over time, especially among non-kin members (e.g., friends, neighbors, congregational members), although some people may prefer limited social networks and occasional solitude (Conway et al. 2013; Finlay and Kobayashi 2018). Others suggest that older Black adults report marginally lower overall loneliness and emotional loneliness, but not social loneliness, than older white adults after controlling for various sociodemographic, cognitive, and psychosocial variables in the Health and Retirement Study (Lee et al. 2022).

The dichotomy between subjective loneliness and objective social isolation has been quantified in Black adults, such that the rate of *objective* social isolation (lack of frequency in contact) from family and friends was one in four but the rate of *subjective* social isolation (lack of perceived closeness) from family and friends was one in six (Taylor et al. 2020). This may suggest that objective social isolation may not always translate into disparities in loneliness. Additionally, Black and white adults do not differ on objective isolation from neighborhoods, from neighborhood groups, from family, and from friends, but white adults are more likely to be isolated from congregational members, more likely to be childless, and more likely to live alone (Taylor et al. 2019). Within Black communities, higher educational attainment may be associated with greater isolation from neighborhood groups, while being female and living in the Southern portion of the United States may be associated with less isolation from congregational members and from family (Taylor et al. 2019). Together, these findings underscore the importance of neighborhood communities, religious congregations, and the family structure in preventing feelings of loneliness and subjective isolation in Black adults, especially given the synergistic effects that positive family networks and congregational networks may have on each other (Nguyen et al. 2016).

Both loneliness and social isolation are dynamic psychological states that vary within and between days. That is, someone may feel lonely in the morning one day but not in the evening, and another person may feel lonely on Monday but not on Tuesday. Because of this, assessing loneliness in "real time" is of great importance. Researchers who have employed ecological momentary assessment (i.e., using technology to assess loneliness in real time) have found no differences in momentary loneliness by race (Compernolle et al. 2021). When further examining the effect on loneliness of being at home, Compernolle et al. (2021) found that being at home was more strongly tied to loneliness among white adults than among Black adults. This may suggest that the family structure of Black adults in the United States (e.g., being less likely to live alone and more likely to live with dependents) (Taylor et al. 2019) may be somewhat protective of loneliness when at home. Given the large and growing demographic of young Black children and adolescents in America (Tamir 2021), many Black adults and older adults may be protected from loneliness when at home.

Social determinants of health may explain any differences in loneliness and social disconnection among Black adults. Hawkley et al. (2008) conducted a study in urban Chicago to better understand the factors that explain loneliness. They found that the higher rate of loneliness found among Black adults in this sample was primarily explained by education and income inequality, which directly influenced proximal factors of loneliness such as health, stress, network size, and marital and social relationship quality. In addition to education and income, gender identity may also influence rates of loneliness among Black adults.

Being a Black woman in the United States comes with aggressive cultural expectations of matriarchal leadership in the face of adversity. The "strong Black woman" schema encouraged by the media and internalized by many successful Black women has previously been associated with worse perceived social support, greater psychological distress, maladaptive perfectionism, low levels of self-compassion, and reduced use of social networks to cope (Liao et al. 2020; Watson-Singleton 2017). As such, it may come as no surprise that loneliness in Black women may be more detrimental to mental and physical health than loneliness in Black men (Chang 2018), and both perfectionism and loneliness may exacerbate depressive and anxious symptoms (Chang 2017). Among HIV-infected Black women, an especially marginalized community, loneliness was also associated with greater illicit drug use and heavier alcohol consumption (Mannes et al. 2016), but this was not true among HIV-infected Black men. This reinforces the dichotomy that strong Black women not only are required by society to be exceptional in the face of adversity but also experience greater distress when they experience loneliness.

Overall, although social disconnection may be greater in Black adults than in white adults, and social networks may decrease over time, it is unclear whether this translates to any difference in loneliness. Moreover, greater loneliness in Black adults may be explained by other social determinants of health in certain samples, such as those residing in urban settings. Research is clearly needed to better understand whether quality of loneliness differs among Black adults and what situations precede feelings of loneliness. Studies have agreed that the social determinants of health, sex, family network, and household structure may influence both social isolation and loneliness in Black adults, as well as the effects of loneliness on health. A vast majority of studies look at loneliness at one time point, and future research should incorporate ecological momentary assessment and longitudinal analyses. Interventions for loneliness and social isolation in the Black population are limited and understudied and are urgently warranted.

Immigrant Community

Immigrants are more likely to report higher levels of loneliness than non-immigrants (Wu and Penning 2015). It has been suggested that longer duration of stay in a given country could lead to improvement in the experience of loneliness of first-generation immigrants (Wu and Penning 2015). Time spent in the country to which one migrated was seen to reduce loneliness in first-generation Portuguese immigrants living in Luxembourg (Albert 2021). However, older age at the time of migration might pose a higher risk for loneliness. For instance, Albert (2021) reported that individuals with greater levels of loneliness were found to be older at the time of immigration. This could be related not only to the shorter length of stay but also to difficulties adapting to a new culture. In contrast, Stick et al. (2021) found that recent and long-staying immigrants living in Canada reported higher levels of loneliness than non-immigrants, with length of stay not positively influencing a decline in levels of loneliness.

Health, family cohesion, and the experience of intergenerational value consensus with one's own children are negatively associated with loneliness in immigrants (Albert 2021). Family conflict was identified as a predictor of loneliness. It is also possible that personality traits influence immigrants' experience of loneliness. For instance, in a study of Chinese older adults living in Chicago, loneliness was positively associated with neuroticism and negatively associated with conscientiousness (Wang and Dong 2018). Factors influencing loneliness included satisfaction with social support and social network size in older Korean women (Kim 1999). In addition, ethnic attachment and functional status predicted loneliness, but marital status did not.

Loneliness also affects international students who migrate to a given country to achieve a goal and might return to their home country after the goal is achieved. African university students living in Portugal reported greater levels of loneliness than non-international students (Neto 2021). Some of the challenges that these students with greater levels of loneliness experienced were related to financial difficulties and perceived discrimination. Factors related to acculturation were also among those influencing loneliness. However, length of stay, age, and gender did not relate to loneliness. Elsewhere, perceived discrimination was also shown to affect loneliness, with those experiencing discrimination reporting higher levels of loneliness (Neto et al. 2017).

There are reports of differences in the experience of loneliness depending on the culture in which an individual lives and one's cultural values of origin (Barreto et al. 2021). For instance, those living in individualist cultures reported greater levels of loneliness than did those living in collectivist cultures. Immigrants undergo a process of *acculturation*, which refers to the process of adapting to the new or dominant culture to which one has migrated. In the process of acculturation, a person may rely on one of four possible strategies: integration, assimilation, separation, and marginalization (Berry et al. 1987). *Integration* refers to when an individual from a minority culture has been able to incorporate several factors of and adapt to the dominant culture. Individuals who use the *assimilation* or *separation* strategies either reject their native or identified culture and value the dominant culture or reject the dominant culture and accept only their native/identified culture. *Marginalization* refers to when individuals identify with neither the dominant culture nor their own culture (Berry et al. 1987).

Research investigating the link between acculturation and loneliness has shown that these acculturation strategies are either positively or negatively associated with loneliness. For instance, second-generation Portuguese students living in Paris with an integration acculturation strategy reported lower levels of loneliness than those with either an assimilation or separation strategy (Neto 2021). Individuals with lower levels of loneliness also had greater life satisfaction, lower levels of stress secondary to acculturation, and less social anxiety. Those employing an integration strategy presented with psychological adaptation and sociocultural adaptation. Similar associations between acculturation strategies and loneliness were found in a study with Brazilian immigrants living in Portugal (Neto et al. 2017). Marginalization was also found to be negatively associated with loneliness. These results suggest that it is best to have opportunities both to maintain ties with one's heritage culture and to establish ties with the host culture.

Immigrants who are more involved in their own culture experience lower levels of loneliness (Sharma 2012). This was found to be true for first- and second-generation immigrants from several countries who were living in the United States. The second generation of immigrants gained information about their native culture from their parents, and this education facilitated their participation in their native culture. First-generation immigrants who were more involved in American culture felt more included but also more lonely; those who were more involved in their native culture felt more discriminated against but less lonely. For the third generation, those who identified with the host culture felt less lonely.

First-generation immigrants may also experience more loneliness than second-generation persons or descendants born in a new country. For example, Arab immigrants living in the United States reported higher levels of loneliness, lower levels of acculturation, and smaller social networks than U.S.-born Arab Americans (Ajrouch 2008). Furthermore, results indicated that acculturation explained immigrant differences in social isolation, whereas loneliness was influenced by marital status.

LGBTQ+ Community

The LGBTQ+ community is a marginalized group in the United States and abroad. Currently, 69 countries around the world have made homosexuality illegal (including the marginalization of queer and trans identities); nearly half of these countries are in Africa. Discrimination toward individuals who identify as LGBTQ+ has been largely influenced by cultural and religious attitudes and misinformation regarding the spread of infectious diseases (e.g., HIV/AIDS). Only in 2015 did the United States legalize same-sex marriage, and in 2021 the U.S. president reversed policies that once barred transgender Americans from enlisting in the armed forces. Progress is being made for barring discrimination against the LGBTQ+ community, although marginalization of varying degrees continues globally.

In 2020, 5.6% of adults identified as LGBTQ+ (55% bisexual, 37% gay or lesbian, 11% transgender, and 3% queer) (Jones 2021). In comparison to the Baby Boomers (born 1946–1964; 2%) and Generation X (born 1965–1980; 4%), Millennials (born 1981–1996; 9%) and Generation Z (born 1997–2002; 16%) are more likely to identify as LGBTQ+ (Jones 2021). Despite a growing share of the population identifying as LGBTQ+ or as an advocate, loneliness remains a significant issue in this population. On average, LGBTQ+ adults are more lonely, depressed, and anxious and have lower perceived social support, greater social isolation, and a higher risk of suicidality than heterosexual cisgender adults (Eres et al. 2021; Fokkema and Kuyper 2009; Haney 2021). Loneliness is estimated to be greater among LGBTQ+ adults, with a medium effect size ($d=0.352$) in a small meta-analysis of four studies (Gorczynski and Fasoli 2021), although the trajectory of loneliness (i.e., change over time) is expected to be equivalent between LGBTQ+ adults and heterosexual cisgender adults (Beam and Collins 2019).

Minority stress theory (Hoy-Ellis and Fredriksen-Goldsen 2016) suggests that LGBTQ+ adults belong to a marginalized community (like ethnic/racial minorities) and, therefore, will experience minority stressors (e.g., discrimination, lack of access, reduced social support) that may ultimately affect their physical and mental health. Note that these minority stressors may compound among LGBTQ+ adults who share other marginalized identities (e.g., being Black or Hispanic/Latinx and identifying as LGBTQ+) (Cyrus 2017; Kim and Fredriksen-Goldsen 2017). Older LGBTQ+ adults are at a higher risk of problematic alcohol consumption (Bryan et al. 2017) and cigarette smoking (Nelson and Andel 2020), as well as having greater multimorbidity (Hoy-Ellis and Fredriksen-Goldsen 2016), perceived stress, worse mental health (Hoy-Ellis and Fredriksen-Goldsen 2016, 2017; Kim and Fredriksen-Goldsen 2017; Nelson and Andel 2020), and greater cognitive decline (Correro and Nielson 2020; Hsieh et al. 2021). Moreover, health services may be inadequate, insensitive, or outwardly prejudiced and discriminatory toward LGBTQ+ adults (de Vries et al. 2019; Sharek et al. 2015; Shnoor and Berg-Warman 2019).

Older LGBTQ+ adults may lack connection within the LGBTQ+ community (Perone et al. 2020), which is associated with social isolation and loneliness (Kneale et al. 2021). Establishing connections with LGBTQ+-specific social groups and other communities with individuals who appreciate, understand, and share similar identities is crucial for LGBTQ+ adults to stave off loneliness and social isolation (Wilkens 2016), especially when family relationships are strained due to their identity (Fokkema and Kuyper 2009; Green 2016).

Social network size is positively associated with employment, income, having a dependent child or partner, being "out" to a neighbor, attending religious organizations, and utilizing LGBTQ+-specific services or programs (Erosheva et al. 2016). Other studies have found that network size and social support are positively associated with physical and mental health–related quality of life among LGBTQ+ adults (Fredriksen-Goldsen et al. 2015), whereas being childless, living alone, not having a partner, being estranged from friends and family, feeling shame, experiencing loss, and having less social embeddedness are associated with greater loneliness among older LGBTQ+ adults (de Guzman et al. 2017; de Vries et al. 2019; Fish and Weis 2019; Fokkema and Kuyper 2009; Mereish and Poteat 2015; Ribeiro-Gonçalves et al. 2022).

In sum, various research study findings suggest that LGBTQ+ adults are lonelier and more socially disconnected in comparison with heterosexual cisgender adults. The difference in loneliness may be due to a complex interaction among internal psychosocial battles (e.g., shame, internalized homophobia), social relationships (e.g., lower social support, smaller networks, estrangement from family and friends, losses), other social determinants of health (e.g., partner/marital status, employment and income, access to adequate health care services), discrimination and prejudice, and both physical and mental health. Research is needed in this marginalized community, including the young and growing population of Millennial and Generation Z adolescents and adults who identify as LGBTQ+. The vast majority of studies look at loneliness at one time point, and future work should incorporate ecological momentary assessment and longitudinal analyses when available. Interventions for loneliness and social isolation in the LGBTQ+ population are limited and understudied.

Case Vignettes

Maria and Jose

Maria, who is 39 years old and from Cuba, has been in a romantic relationship for 6 years with Jose, who is 42 years old and from Argentina. Maria has been living in the United States for 15 years and Jose for about 7 years. Jose's siblings live in the same town as Jose and Maria. Maria's immediate and extended family are in Cuba, and she sends them money on a monthly basis. Maria is fluent in Spanish and understands English but only partly. Jose is fluent in both English and Spanish. They have a 6-year-old son, Carlos, who has academic performance difficulties. Carlos is fluent in English and understands Spanish but does not respond to conversations in Spanish, although he could. Maria and Jose are seeking couples counseling after Jose was diagnosed with a cardiovascular disease and depression.

What might be some factors to assess when you meet with Jose and Maria?

In addition to considering the biopsychosocial model when discussing symptoms and life experiences, it is important to assess for negative life events, acculturation, perceived discrimination, loneliness and social isolation, other mental health symptoms, social network and social support system(s), spirituality, quality of life, eating habits, suicidality, and hopelessness, as well as specific cultural values and beliefs because Maria and Jose are from different countries. You might also want to ask questions about their routine at home and consider discussing therapy for their son or family.

What might be some considerations to make when providing services to Jose and Maria?

When considering working with Jose and Maria, you may want to be culturally sensitive and gain more knowledge about their respective cultures. If you are not culturally competent and are not able to gain competence or receive supervision from someone who is, you might want to consider referring Maria and Jose to providers who are.

What interventions would you consider?

There are different interventions to consider in this scenario. For instance, you might want to ask for permission (verbal and written) to contact and work with the medical provider in order to learn more about Jose's medical condition and collaborate on interventions. It also is important to assess Maria's and Jose's knowledge of depression, cardiovascular conditions, and other topics discussed and to provide psychoeducation on different topics (e.g., the association between cardiovascular conditions and depression/other symptoms, acculturation). You might also want to encourage them to increase social support by connecting with neighbors, work colleagues, and others with whom they can establish relationships or by volunteering or attending community events. Meanwhile, you want to assess possible obstacles to social participation and brainstorm solutions with them.

Referrals to discuss with Maria and Jose include 1) seeing a social worker who might be able to connect them with local resources, including English classes for Maria, 2) individual therapy for Jose and child psychotherapy for their son, Carlos, and 3) family therapy. After discussing the pros and cons of different interventions, invite Maria and Jose to join you in deciding which intervention(s) they want to pursue.

Donna

Donna is a 68-year-old Black woman who is cognitively intact and functionally independent. She worked for 40 years as an elementary school teacher in a suburb of Atlanta, Georgia. On her 65th birthday, Donna and her husband, Michael, sold their Atlanta home and moved into a condo in Savannah to be closer in proximity to their two adult children. Donna is recently widowed after losing Michael to stage 4 colorectal cancer after 42 years of marriage. She is financially stable and spends most of her time volunteering at a community church, hosting weekend camps for young children with intellectual disabilities. Beyond her volunteering duties, Donna occasionally babysits her six grandchildren. Nothing makes Donna happier than volunteering and spending time with her grandchildren.

However, when Donna is home alone, she often finds herself feeling lonely and socially disconnected from her neighborhood. Donna compulsively ruminates over Michael's death when she feels lonely, longing for the life that she and Michael had planned together for decades. When Donna and Michael moved to Savannah, they did not anticipate how racially divided their new community would be. Although Donna has not experienced overt prejudice or discrimination from her white neighbors, she has little in common with them and therefore limits her socializing to church and family. Donna was recently asked by her primary care physician whether she was depressed after he learned that Michael had recently passed away, to which she responded by strongly denying any depression. Uncomfortable, the primary care physician quickly moved to Donna's physical assessment without another question about her psychosocial well-being.

What context has the physician lost by not inquiring about Donna's family interactions and social well-being?

If the physician had asked Donna about her social well-being, her loneliness would have been uncovered and a treatment plan could have been discussed, even if she ultimately denied a need for treatment.

What might be a treatment plan for Donna's loneliness?

The literature suggests that one protective factor of loneliness in Black adults may be family interaction within the home. Seeing this, a clinician could encourage Donna to reach out to her adult children. Babysitting more often may reduce her loneliness and her adult children's stress levels. Additionally, the clinician may encourage Donna to reach out to the social networks that she has cultivated at church, including spending time outside of the church itself in community neighborhoods in which she feels comfortable and supported.

Samuel

Samuel is a single 56-year-old Latinx man who identifies as queer and bisexual and uses "he/him" gender pronouns. He grew up in the Bronx, New York City, and works as a project manager for a Fortune 500 company. For most of his life, Samuel has had to hide who he really is from his work colleagues and family. Growing up, he was ridiculed by his classmates for showing a sexual interest in men and learned that being bisexual or identifying as queer was not widely accepted in the Catholic church. Occasionally, he would receive beatings from his father and uncles if he did not dress in line with his family's values. Many things positively changed in Samuel's life when he left the Bronx for an undergraduate education. When Samuel entered university, he found a community of LGBTQ+ individuals who accepted him for who he was. However, his university experience was not entirely positive. Samuel lost a considerable number of friends to the HIV/ AIDS epidemic and found it difficult to obtain employment upon graduation. Although he could never prove that discrimination led to his unemployment, it did seem relevant. Once Samuel began to dress differently and change his mannerisms in corporate America, he was successful in obtaining a well-paying job in Manhattan.

Now, 30 years later, Samuel has the job that he dreamed of, but his social life is strained. He has strong connections within the drag community of New York City, but most of these relationships are superficial. Outside of performance art, Samuel has difficulty maintaining long-lasting friendships and has never been partnered for longer than 2 years. Although he is surrounded by like-minded friends who are supportive of his gender identity and sexual preference, Samuel worries that his age has affected his chance at intimate or meaningful friendships. Indeed, many of Samuel's friends are considerably younger and grew up in an era in which gender and sexual fluidity were better articulated and captured in the media and the urban population. This detachment from friends and a distinct lack of similarly aged connections has caused Samuel to develop feelings of severe loneliness, even when among others.

What has contributed to Samuel's loneliness?

Samuel identifies as Latinx and LGBTQ+ and is part of a birth cohort in which gender and sexual minorities were disproportionately affected by the HIV/AIDS epidemic in the United States. He has likely been subject to hiring discrimination and has limited meaningful contact with his family due to polarized belief systems. Although he developed a strong social network of like-minded individuals in the LGBTQ+ community, he feels "out of place" in Manhattan due to his age and his lack of ability to initiate deeper connections.

How might a clinician improve Samuel's social well-being?

Samuel does not experience significant social isolation but does feel lonely. This suggests that although he is surrounded by others, he has a distinct negative appraisal of the situation that leads to feelings of loneliness. Addressing his appraisal of social situations and the relationships that he has formed may improve Samuel's well-being. Perhaps others in his community do not view age as a barrier to developing deeper connections with Samuel; this perception may be one that Samuel has created and is maintaining as a self-fulfilling prophecy. Psychotherapy may be necessary to discuss whether the considerable loss that Samuel suffered while at university has contributed to his attachment style as a middle-aged adult. A clinician may not be able to improve family relations, so focusing on the network that Samuel has developed will be crucial.

Recommendations for Future Work

More research is needed to address inconsistent findings from different studies, which may be the result of the use of different measures, over- versus underreporting of symptoms, and varied levels of underrepresentation of different races/ethnicities. Future studies should encourage more intragroup racial/ethnic investigations in loneliness-related research to understand heterogeneity among groups, highlighting the differential influence of determinants of health across group members. This is especially true for Hispanic/Latinx groups in the United States because much of this work entirely disregards the within-group heterogeneity masked by the label of Hispanic/Latinx ethnicity, failing to discern any differences between ethnicities such as Mexican, Puerto Rican, Central American, and Cuban (Pérez and Ailshire 2017; Shor et al. 2017), all of whom would have a unique immigration, discrimination, and acculturation experience in the United States. The generalizability of study results is, therefore, often limited for racial/ethnic subgroups. Additionally, much of the research that examines loneliness among racial/ethnic, gender, and sexual minorities does so in comparison with white groups, positioning white persons as the gold standard in the measurement and reporting of all health and social outcomes. As population demographics in the United States shift, with current racial/ethnic minority groups becoming the majority, referring to white persons as the uniform reference group may need to be qualified (Brown and Tucker-Seeley 2018). Finally, results usually reflect cross-sectional data, limiting analysis and interpretation regarding causality. Self-report has its own set of limitations as well.

Considering the ramifications of loneliness and social isolation for one's mental and physical health, multilevel interventions and policy changes are needed. Interventions that promote social support and acceptance are warranted. A peer-support intervention provided relief in the experience of loneliness in Chinese participants who migrated to Canada (Lai et al. 2020). There is evidence that shared-identity social support groups are effective in reducing loneliness among ethnic minority groups. A series of interventions to reduce loneliness among minority ethnic groups are reviewed by Salway et al. (2020).

These findings call for attention to the differences in how loneliness might be experienced by and affect Hispanic/Latinx individuals and immigrants of other races/ethnicities. It is important to be aware of immigration history as well as the acculturation processes experienced by a person as an individual and as a part of a group. Thus, public policies and mental health professionals should address the different needs of immigrants and their descendants in a manner that is sensitive to their backgrounds and promotes social integration and support.

KEY POINTS

- Loneliness is common among marginalized communities of Hispanic/Latinx, Black, immigrant, and LGBTQ+ individuals.

- Immigrants are at a higher risk of experiencing loneliness than non-immigrants.

- It is important to assess for and address acculturation strategies and perceived discrimination because these are likely to contribute to the experience of loneliness.

- Marginalized groups commonly face health and health care inequities, and clinicians must focus on ensuring access to necessary community resources.

Suggested Readings

Barreto M, Victor C, Hammond C, et al: Loneliness around the world: age, gender, and cultural differences in loneliness. Pers Individ Dif 169:110066, 2021 33536694

Cross WE Jr, Vandiver BJ: Nigrescence theory and measurement: introducing the Cross Racial Identity Scale (CRIS), in Handbook of Multicultural Counseling, 2nd Edition. Edited by Ponerotto JG, Casas JM, Suzuki LM, Alexander CM. Thousand Oaks, CA, Sage, 2001, pp 371–393

Sue DW, Sue D: Counseling the Culturally Diverse: Theory and Practice, 4th Edition. New York, John Wiley, 2003

References

Ajrouch KJ: Social isolation and loneliness among Arab American elders: cultural, social, and personal factors. Res Hum Dev 5(1):44–59, 2008

Albert I: Perceived loneliness and the role of cultural and intergenerational belonging: the case of Portuguese first-generation immigrants in Luxembourg. Eur J Ageing 18(3):299–310, 2021 34483795

Alberti FB: A Biography of Loneliness: The History of an Emotion. New York, Oxford University Press, 2019

Ansion M, Merali N: Latino immigrant parents' experiences raising young children in the absence of extended family networks in Canada: implications for counseling. Couns Psychol Q 31(4):408–427, 2018

Barreto M, Victor C, Hammond C, et al: Loneliness around the world: age, gender, and cultural differences in loneliness. Pers Individ Dif 169:110066, 2021 33536694

Beam CR, Collins EM: Trajectories of depressive symptomatology and loneliness in older adult sexual minorities and heterosexual groups. Clin Gerontol 42(2):172–184, 2019 30321105

Berry JW, Kim U, Minde T, Monk D: Comparative studies of acculturative stress. Int Migr Rev 21:491–511, 1987

Brown L, Tucker-Seeley R: Commentary: will "deaths of despair" among whites change how we talk about racial/ethnic health disparities? Ethn Dis 28(2):123–128, 2018 29725197

Bryan AE, Kim HJ, Fredriksen-Goldsen KI: Factors associated with high-risk alcohol consumption among LGB older adults: the roles of gender, social support, perceived stress, discrimination, and stigma. Gerontologist 57(suppl 1):S95–S104, 2017 28087799

Cacioppo JT, Cacioppo S: Loneliness in the modern age: an evolutionary theory of loneliness (ETL). Adv Exp Soc Psychol 58:127–197, 2018

Caplan S: Latinos, acculturation, and acculturative stress: a dimensional concept analysis. Policy Polit Nurs Pract 8(2):93–106, 2007 17652627

Chang EC: Perfectionism and loneliness as predictors of depressive and anxious symptoms in African American adults: further evidence for a top-down additive model. Cognit Ther Res 41(5):720–729, 2017

Chang EC: Relationship between loneliness and symptoms of anxiety and depression in African American men and women: evidence for gender as a moderator. Pers Individ Dif 120:138–143, 2018

Chang EC, Díaz L, Lucas AG, et al: Ethnic identity and loneliness in predicting suicide risk in Latino college students. Hisp J Behav Sci 39(4):470–485, 2017

Chetty R, Hendren N, Jones MR, Porter SR: Race and economic opportunity in the United States: an intergenerational perspective. Q J Econ 135(2):711–783, 2020

Compernolle EL, Finch LE, Hawkley LC, Cagney KA: Momentary loneliness among older adults: contextual difference and their moderation by gender and race/ethnicity. Soc Sci Med 285:114307, 2021 34375898

Conway F, Magai C, Jones S, et al: A six-year follow-up study of social network changes among African-American, Caribbean, and U.S.-born Caucasian urban older adults. Int J Aging Hum Dev 76(1):1–27, 2013 23540157

Cornwell B, Laumann EO, Schumm LP: The social connectedness of older adults: a national profile. Am Sociol Rev 73(2):185–203, 2008 19018292

Correro AN 2nd, Nielson KA: A review of minority stress as a risk factor for cognitive decline in lesbian, gay, bisexual, and transgender (LGBT) elders. J Gay Lesbian Ment Health 24(1):2–19, 2020 33014237

Cyrus K: Multiple minorities as multiply marginalized: applying the minority stress theory to LGBTQ people of color. J Gay Lesbian Ment Health 21(3):194–202, 2017

de Guzman AB, Valdez LP, Orpiana MB, et al: Against the current: a grounded theory study on the estrangement experiences of a select group of Filipino gay older persons. Educ Gerontol 43(7):329–340, 2017

de Vries B, Gutman G, Humble Á, et al: End-of-life preparations among LGBT older Canadian adults: the missing conversations. Int J Aging Hum Dev 88(4):358–379, 2019 30871331

Dominguez-Fuentes JM, Hombrados-Mendieta MI: Social support and happiness in immigrant women in Spain. Psychol Rep 110(3):977–990, 2012 22897099

Eres R, Postolovski N, Thielking M, Lim MH: Loneliness, mental health, and social health indicators in LGBTQIA+ Australians. Am J Orthopsychiatry 91(3):358–366, 2021 33315419

Erosheva EA, Kim HJ, Emlet C, Fredriksen-Goldsen KI: Social networks of lesbian, gay, bisexual, and transgender older adults. Res Aging 38(1):98–123, 2016 25882129

Finlay JM, Kobayashi LC: Social isolation and loneliness in later life: a parallel convergent mixed-methods case study of older adults and their residential contexts in the Minneapolis metropolitan area, USA. Soc Sci Med 208:25–33, 2018 29758475

Fish J, Weis C: All the lonely people, where do they all belong? An interpretive synthesis of loneliness and social support in older lesbian, gay and bisexual communities. Qual Ageing Older Adults 2019 Epub ahead of print

Fisher FD, Reitzel LR, Nguyen N, et al: Loneliness and self-rated health among church-attending African Americans. Am J Health Behav 38(4):481–491, 2014 24636110

Fokkema T, Kuyper L: The relation between social embeddedness and loneliness among older lesbian, gay, and bisexual adults in the Netherlands. Arch Sex Behav 38(2):264–275, 2009 18034297

Foti SA, Khambaty T, Birnbaum-Weitzman O, et al: Loneliness, cardiovascular disease, and diabetes prevalence in the Hispanic community health study/study of Latinos sociocultural ancillary study. J Immigr Minor Health 22(2):345–352, 2020 30963348

Fredriksen-Goldsen KI, Kim HJ, Shiu C, et al: Successful aging among LGBT older adults: physical and mental health-related quality of life by age group. Gerontologist 55(1):154–168, 2015 25213483

Gallegos ML, Segrin C: Exploring the mediating role of loneliness in the relationship between spirituality and health: implications for the Latino health paradox. Psychology of Religion and Spirituality 11(3):308–318, 2019

Gerst-Emerson K, Shovali TE, Markides KS: Loneliness among very old Mexican Americans: findings from the Hispanic Established Populations Epidemiologic Studies of the Elderly. Arch Gerontol Geriatr 59(1):145–149, 2014 24582944

Gorczynski P, Fasoli F: Loneliness in sexual minority and heterosexual individuals: a comparative meta-analysis. Journal of Gay and Lesbian Mental Health 1–18, 2021

Green M: Do the companionship and community networks of older LGBT adults compensate for weaker kinship networks? Qual Ageing Older Adults 17(1):36–49, 2016

Hamilton D, Darity W Jr, Price AE, et al: Umbrellas Don't Make It Rain: Why Studying and Working Hard Isn't Enough for Black Americans. New York, The New School, 2015, pp 780–781

Haney JL: Suicidality risk among adult sexual minorities: results from a cross-sectional population-based survey. J Gay Lesbian Soc Serv 33(2):250–271, 2021

Hawkley LC, Hughes ME, Waite LJ, et al: From social structural factors to perceptions of relationship quality and loneliness: the Chicago Health, Aging, and Social Relations Study. J Gerontol B Psychol Sci Soc Sci 63(6):S375–S384, 2008 19092047

Hawkley LC, Thisted RA, Masi CM, Cacioppo JT: Loneliness predicts increased blood pressure: 5-year cross-lagged analyses in middle-aged and older adults. Psychol Aging 25(1):132–141, 2010 20230134

Heredia D Jr, Gonzalez MLS, Rosner CM, et al: The influence of loneliness and interpersonal relations on Latina/o middle school students' wellbeing. Journal of Latinos and Education 16(4):338–348, 2017

Holt-Lunstad J, Smith TB, Baker M, et al: Loneliness and social isolation as risk factors for mortality: a meta-analytic review. Perspect Psychol Sci 10(2):227–237, 2015 25910392

Hoy-Ellis CP, Fredriksen-Goldsen KI: Depression among transgender older adults: general and minority stress. Am J Community Psychol 59(3–4):295–305, 2017 28369987

Hoy-Ellis CP, Fredriksen-Goldsen KI: Lesbian, gay, and bisexual older adults: linking internal minority stressors, chronic health conditions, and depression. Aging Ment Health 20(11):1119–1130, 2016 27050776

Hurtado-de-Mendoza A, Gonzales FA, Serrano A, Kaltman S: Social isolation and perceived barriers to establishing social networks among Latina immigrants. Am J Community Psychol 53(1–2):73–82, 2014 24402726

Hsieh N, Liu H, Lai WH: Elevated risk of cognitive impairment among older sexual minorities: Do health conditions, health behaviors, and social connections matter? Gerontologist 61(3):352–362, 2021 32951038

Jeste DV, Lee EE, Cacioppo S: Battling the modern behavioral epidemic of loneliness: suggestions for research and interventions. JAMA Psychiatry 77(6):553–554, 2020 32129811

Jones JM: LGBT identification rises to 5.6% in latest U.S. estimates. Gallup, February 24, 2021. Available at: https://news.gallup.com/poll/329708/lgbt-identification-rises-latest-estimate.aspx. Accessed October 26, 2021.

Kim HJ, Fredriksen-Goldsen KI: Disparities in mental health quality of life between Hispanic and non-Hispanic white LGB midlife and older adults and the influence of lifetime discrimination, social connectedness, socioeconomic status, and perceived stress. Res Aging 39(9):991–1012, 2017 27193047

Kim O: Predictors of loneliness in elderly Korean immigrant women living in the United States of America. J Adv Nurs 29(5):1082–1088, 1999 10320490

Kneale D, Henley J, Thomas J, French R: Inequalities in older LGBT people's health and care needs in the United Kingdom: a systematic scoping review. Ageing Soc 41(3):493–515, 2021 34531622

Lai DWL, Li J, Ou X, Li CYP: Effectiveness of a peer-based intervention on loneliness and social isolation of older Chinese immigrants in Canada: a randomized controlled trial. BMC Geriatr 20(1):356, 2020 32958076

Lee J, Hong J, Zhou Y, Robles G: The relationships between loneliness, social support, and resilience among Latinx immigrants in the United States. Clin Soc Work J 48(1):99–109, 2020 33583968

Lee JH, Luchetti M, Aschwanden D, et al: Cognitive impairment and the trajectory of loneliness in older adulthood: evidence from the Health and Retirement Study. J Aging Health 34(1):3–13, 2022 34027689

Liao KYH, Wei M, Yin M: The misunderstood schema of the strong Black woman: exploring its mental health consequences and coping responses among African American women. Psychol Women Q 44(1):84–104, 2020

Mannes ZL, Burrell LE, Bryant VE, et al: Loneliness and substance use: the influence of gender among HIV+ Black/African American adults 50+. AIDS care 28(5):598–602, 2016

Martinez IL, Baron AC, Largaespada V, et al: Social correlates of depressive symptoms among Cuban and other Latino older adults in South Florida. J Cult Divers 26(4):149–156, 2019

Mereish EH, Poteat VP: A relational model of sexual minority mental and physical health: the negative effects of shame on relationships, loneliness, and health. J Couns Psychol 62(3):425–437, 2015 26010289

Nelson CL, Andel R: Does sexual orientation relate to health and well-being? Analysis of adults 50+ years of age. Gerontologist 60(7):1282–1290, 2020 31909416

Neto F: Loneliness among African international students at Portuguese universities. Journal of International Students 11(2):397–416, 2021

Neto J, Nazaré E, Neto F: Acculturation, adaptation and loneliness among Brazilian migrants living in Portugal, in People's Movements in the 21st Century: Risks, Challenges, and Benefits. Edited by Muenstermann I. Rijeka, Croatia, InTech, 2017, pp 169–185

Nguyen AW, Chatters LM, Taylor RJ: African American extended family and church-based social network typologies. Fam Relat 65(5):701–715, 2016 28479650

Noe-Bustamante L, Flores A: Facts on Latinos in the U.S. Pew Research Center, September 16, 2019. Available at: www.pewresearch.org/hispanic/fact-sheet/latinos-in-the-u-s-fact-sheet. Accessed October 26, 2021.

Parsai M, Nieri T, Perreira K, et al: Becoming an American parent: overcoming challenges and finding strength in a new immigrant Latino community. J Fam Issues 27:1383–1414, 2006

Pérez C, Ailshire JA: Aging in Puerto Rico: a comparison of health status among island Puerto Rican and mainland U.S. older adults. J Aging Health 29(6):1056–1078, 2017 28599584 Epub ahead of print

Perone AK, Ingersoll-Dayton B, Watkins-Dukhie K: Social isolation loneliness among LGBT older adults: lessons learned from a pilot friendly caller program. Clinical Social Work Journal 48(1):126-139, 2020

Perreira K, Chapman M, Stein G: Becoming an American parent: overcoming challenges and finding strength in a new immigrant Latino community. Journal of Family Issues 27:1383–1414, 2006

Ribeiro-Gonçalves JA, Pereira H, Costa PA, et al: Loneliness, social support, and adjustment to aging in older Portuguese gay men. Sexuality Research and Social Policy 19(5), 2022

Salway S, Such E, Preston L, et al: Reducing loneliness among migrant and ethnic minority people: a participatory evidence synthesis. Public Health Res 8(10):1–246, 2020

Sharek DB, McCann E, Sheerin F, et al: Older LGBT people's experiences and concerns with healthcare professionals and services in Ireland. Int J Older People Nurs 10(3):230–240, 2015 25418672

Sharma R: The relationship between loneliness, ethnic identity, and dimensions of membership across first, second, and third generation Americans. Colonial Academic Alliance Undergraduate Research Journal 3(9), 2012

Shiovitz-Ezra S, Parag O: Does loneliness "get under the skin"? Associations of loneliness with subsequent change in inflammatory and metabolic markers. Aging Ment Health 23(10):1358–1366, 2019 30380911

Shnoor Y, Berg-Warman A: Needs of the aging LGBT community in Israel. Int J Aging Hum Dev 89(1):77–92, 2019 31032619

Shor E, Roelfs D, Vang ZM: The "Hispanic mortality paradox" revisited: meta-analysis and meta-regression of life-course differentials in Latin American and Caribbean immigrants' mortality. Soc Sci Med 186:20–33, 2017 28577458

Stick M, Hon F, Kaida L: Self-reported loneliness among recent immigrants, long-term immigrants, and Canadian-born individuals. Economic and Social Reports 1(7): 2021

Sue DW, Sue D: Counseling the Culturally Diverse: Theory and Practice, 7th Edition. Hoboken, NJ, John Wiley and Sons, 2016

Tamir C: The growing diversity of Black America. Pew Research Center, March 25, 2021. Available at: www.pewresearch.org/social-trends/2021/03/25/the-growing-diversity-of-black-america. Accessed October 26, 2021.

Taylor RJ, Chatters LM, Taylor HO: Race and objective social isolation: older African Americans, black Caribbeans, and non-Hispanic whites. J Gerontol B Psychol Sci Soc 74(8):1429–1440, 2019 30289494

Taylor RJ, Taylor HO, Nguyen AW, Chatters LM: Social isolation from family and friends and mental health among African Americans and Black Caribbeans. Am J Orthopsychiatry 90(4):468–478, 2020 32309977

Tomaka J, Thompson S, Palacios R: The relation of social isolation, loneliness, and social support to disease outcomes among the elderly. J Aging Health 18(3):359–384, 2006 16648391

Villar P: Away from home: paradoxes of parenting for Mexican immigrant adults. Fam Soc 91:201–208, 2010

Watson-Singleton NN: Strong Black woman schema and psychological distress: the mediating role of perceived emotional support. J Black Psychol 43(8):778–788, 2017

Wang B, Dong X: The association between personality and loneliness: findings from a community-dwelling Chinese aging population. Gerontol Geriatr Med 4, 2018 30035191

Wilkens J: The significance of affinity groups and safe spaces for older lesbians and bisexual women: creating support networks and resisting heteronormativity in older age. Qual Ageing Older Adults 17(1):26–35, 2016

Wippold GM, Tucker CM, Roncoroni J, Henry MA: Impact of stress and loneliness on health-related quality of life among low income senior African Americans. J Racial Ethn Health Disparities 8(4):1089–1097, 2021 32940896

Wu Z, Penning M: Immigration and loneliness in later life. Ageing Soc 35(1):64–69, 2015

6

Neurobiology of Loneliness

Jeffrey A. Lam, B.A.
Ellen E. Lee, M.D.

HUMANS ARE A SOCIAL SPECIES, and the absence of quality relationships threatens health and reproductive success (Cacioppo et al. 2014). Humans are believed to have ingrained neural, hormonal, and genetic mechanisms to help navigate social structures and feelings of loneliness. The Cacioppo evolutionary theory of loneliness (Cacioppo and Cacioppo 2018) hypothesizes that loneliness is part of an early biological distress signal to the body that encourages adaptive behavioral changes that help humans increase evolutionary fitness.

In recent years, loneliness has received increasing attention from researchers and has been described as a modern behavioral pandemic, a "chronic disease," a silent killer, and a grand challenge for society (Klinenberg 2018; National Academies of Sciences, Engineering, and Medicine 2020). Researchers define loneliness as a *subjective* feeling of distress due to a discrepancy between desired and perceived social connectedness. This contrasts with *social isolation*, which is defined as the *objective* lack of social contact. Although commonly seen as a psychological reflection of a lack of social relationships, loneliness is a complex, multidimensional construct that is being increasingly linked to biological processes and consequences.

There is evidence that loneliness is associated with dysregulation of numerous biological systems. Several of these findings are reviewed in other chapters of this book. Briefly, there is evidence of relationships between loneliness and cardiovascular disorders (Valtorta et al. 2016), dementia (Kuiper et al. 2015), and mental health outcomes such as anxiety, depression, and suicidal ideation (Beutel et al. 2017). Loneliness and mental illness is reviewed in Chapter 4 ("Loneliness in People Living With Mental Health Disorders"), while "Loneliness Across the Life Span" (including cognitive changes) is reviewed in Chapter 3. On a molecular level, one meta-analysis found loneliness to be associated with higher inflammatory marker levels (Smith et al. 2020) and differential physiological expression toward acute stress situations (Brown et al. 2018). In a widely cited review, Hawkley and Cacioppo (2010) noted consistent differences in the hypothalamic-pituitary-adrenal axis, gene expression, and immune functioning as potential mechanisms for increased morbidity and mortality in lonely individuals. The "Systemic Neuroendocrine and Inflammatory Mechanisms in Loneliness" are reviewed in Chapter 7.

Given its integration with biological processes, loneliness is also a major risk factor for morbidity and mortality, with effects accumulating over time (Hawkley and Cacioppo 2010). Loneliness is associated with a 26% increased likelihood of mortality, independent of one's lifestyle (e.g., smoking, physical activity) and psychological factors (e.g., depression, anxiety) (Holt-Lunstad et al. 2015). Three meta-analyses have found that loneliness is associated with increased all-cause mortality (Holt-Lunstad et al. 2015; Rico-Uribe et al. 2018; Steptoe et al. 2013).

Furthermore, genetics may have a role in the experience of loneliness. Twin studies have estimated the heritability of loneliness to be between 37% and 55%, although molecular genetic studies have not consistently identified any candidate genes that are significantly associated with loneliness after statistical corrections for multiple comparisons (Gao et al. 2017). A recent 2019 study created polygenic risk scores for loneliness that found overlapping risk with cardiovascular, psychiatric, and metabolic disorders (Abdellaoui et al. 2019).

Loneliness and the Brain

Given the rising interest in empirical loneliness research, it is critical to understand the neurobiology of loneliness, a topic that has been less studied until recently. Diagnostically, appreciating the neuroscience of loneliness may help us objectively identify loneliness. Translationally, a better comprehension of the neural underpinnings of loneliness may allow scientists to better conceptualize mental disorders related to social motivation and social cognition, such as autism spectrum disorder, social anxiety disorder, and schizophrenia. Therapeutically, understanding the lonely brain may allow investigators to design interventions to alleviate loneliness, with the goal of reducing overall morbidity and mortality. Chapter 8 ("Interventions for Loneliness in Younger People"), Chapter 9 ("Interventions for Loneliness in Older Adults"), and Chapter 10 ("Community-Based Interventions for Loneliness") review interventions for loneliness.

This chapter aims to review the current literature linking neurobiological findings to loneliness, using the evolutionary theory of loneliness as a framework for discussion. The first section of this chapter creates a picture of the current literature, organized by the neuroimaging methodologies. The last section summarizes the findings and suggests which regions of the brain are most likely to be associated with loneliness.

Overview of Primary Literature

In this section, we summarize the most current literature on the differences between lonely and non-lonely brains. A recent systematic review identified all the literature reports analyzing the relationship between loneliness and neurobiology (Lam et al. 2021). The studies included in the review used a validated loneliness scale, most often the UCLA Loneliness Scale (UCLA LS). Neurobiology measures included assessments of brain structure or function: CT, MRI, functional MRI (fMRI), diffusion tensor imaging (DTI), PET, electroencephalography, and pathology and genetic studies that directly extracted RNA from the brain.

Neuroanatomy

A recent review identified 15 studies that analyzed the relationship between loneliness and neuroanatomy (Lam et al. 2021). Most of these studies used structural MRI to analyze the whole brain and determine which regions of the brain had significantly higher or lower gray or white matter in lonely individuals.

Gray Matter Neuroanatomy

Most of the studies examined gray matter structures in the brain, which are the parts of the brain that primarily consist of cell bodies. Kanai et al. (2012) reported a significant correlation between loneliness and brain structure using a technique called voxel-based morphometry to show that lonely individuals had lower gray matter volume in the left posterior superior temporal sulcus (pSTS), a region thought to process social information (Barbey et al. 2013). Looking for correlations in the whole brain between loneliness and gray matter volume, the authors used a corrected *P* value to control for multiple comparisons.

Using similar methodologies, multiple later studies found a link between loneliness and gray matter of the dorsolateral prefrontal cortex (dlPFC), a part of the prefrontal cortex (PFC) implicated in working memory, executive functioning, and emotional processing (Düzel et al. 2019). One study found that loneliness was positively associated with gray matter volume of the dlPFC, a relationship mediated by the personality traits of neuroticism and extraversion. Another study found that loneliness had a mediating effect on the relationship between dlPFC volume and attitudes toward suicide. Collectively, these studies give evidence that loneliness and personality factors overlap and are associated with differences in regional brain volumes.

Other studies have found correlations between loneliness and the left amygdala, left striatum (left putamen, left caudate, and left pallidum), and cerebellum in loneliness. However, many of these earlier studies were limited by small sample sizes and insufficient control for confounding variables, such as psychopathology, personality factors, and social network characteristics.

In 2019, Düzel and colleagues conducted a study of 319 older adults to attempt to bring more clarity to previous findings. First, they examined the whole brain to find the correlates of individuals high in loneliness, finding that loneliness was associated with smaller gray matter volumes in the left amygdala/anterior hippocampus, left posterior parahippocampus, and left cerebellum. They also confirmed some of the previous neurocorrelates of loneliness by specifically examining the hippocampus and amygdala using a region-of-interest approach. They attempted to control for well-known correlates, such as age and depressive symptoms. The authors found a significant loneliness-by-age interaction for the amygdala and hippocampus and a significant loneliness-by-depression interaction for the nucleus accumbens (Düzel et al. 2019).

White Matter Neuroanatomy

Similarly, other research groups have tried to examine the white matter correlates of loneliness. White matter volume primarily consists of myelinated axons. These studies employed DTI, an MRI imaging technique used to evaluate white matter integrity. Similarly, most analyzed the whole brain to try to find which white matter regions were correlated with loneliness, correcting for multiple comparisons. The studies identified numerous white matter tracts that were significantly associated with loneliness: the bilateral superior longitudinal fasciculus, right anterior insula, left pSTS, left posterior temporoparietal junction, dorsomedial PFC (dmPFC), and left rostrolateral PFC, among other regions.

Other Neuroanatomy Studies

Other studies examined differences in brain structure over time. Cristofori et al. (2019) used voxel-based lesion symptom mapping to examine veterans with penetrating traumatic brain injury in different regions of the brain and how it influenced their perceptions of loneliness 40–45 years post-injury. They found that participants with lesions in the right anterior insula and right PFC were more likely to have *lower* perceptions of loneliness. These results suggest that the insula and right PFC are key regions in the perception of loneliness.

In one of the first intervention studies, Ehlers et al. (2017) found that a 6-month exercise intervention decreased loneliness but was not related to structural changes in the brain. These authors did find that baseline amygdala and PFC volumes moderated the effect of exercise on loneliness over the course of the intervention, giving some evidence that brain structure may predispose some individuals to loneliness. The authors suggested that 6 months may not be long enough to detect changes in the brain structure related to improvements in loneliness.

Another study examined the progression of white matter hyperintensities in the brains of older adult participants for an average of 5.2 years (Duan et al. 2017). They found that those who did not have children in their homes (i.e., empty nest–related psychological distress) and were lonely were more likely to have a progression of white matter lesions during the later phases of the study.

Although structural brain studies have provided early evidence of regional brain differences between lonely and non-lonely individuals, causality cannot be determined because most of the literature is cross-sectional. Furthermore, many of these studies were whole-brain analyses without a priori hypotheses, so the results must be interpreted with caution. Many of these studies have yet to be replicated given the differences in sample characteristics, and these studies also need to control for established confounding variables such as social isolation, depression, and age. Lastly, differences in gray matter regions cannot imply functionality of that given region. Even with these limitations, there is strong evidence of neuroanatomical differences between lonely and non-lonely brains.

Task-Based Studies

A recent review found 10 studies that analyzed the relationship between loneliness and a task-based fMRI paradigm and 3 studies using electroencephalography (Lam et al. 2021). These studies examined brain activity in lonely and non-lonely individuals during experimental tasks, such as looking at positive versus negative social images and positive and negative social words.

fMRI studies have adequate spatial resolution and can identify differences in brain activation when presented with alternative stimuli in an experimental paradigm. Electroencephalographic studies provide better temporal resolution and can provide better evidence of how quickly different regions of the brain react to different stimuli.

Task-Based Functional MRI Studies

Most of the literature with task-based fMRI has attempted to understand differences in brain activation in lonely versus non-lonely individuals in response to positive and negative social stimuli and non-social stimuli. This methodology allows the close examination of discrete social processes that contribute to (or underlie) complex social and emotional functioning or socioemotional function.

In one of the first task-based fMRI studies, Cacioppo et al. (2009) found that lonely individuals showed decreased activation of the ventral striatum, a key region in motivation, compared with non-lonely individuals in response to pleasant social images. This suggests that loneliness may be associated with decreased social approach motivation. Moreover, lonely individuals showed increased visual cortex activation when presented with unpleasant social images, giving evidence that lonely individuals may be more sensitive to negative social cues compared with non-lonely individuals.

In another well-designed study, college students ($N=40$) who were undergoing 10 hours of social isolation or fasting from food had similar activation of the substantia nigra/ventral tegmental area (SN/VTA) (Tomova et al. 2020). Similar to the ventral striatum, this area is also associated with the reward system. This study gave additional evidence that loneliness is a state that alters our desire for social interaction, much like hunger. Interestingly, participants with higher baseline trait UCLA LS scores showed decreased activation in the SN/VTA compared with non-lonely individuals, which may be consistent with the idea that chronic loneliness is associated with social withdrawal.

Two other studies failed to replicate the Cacioppo results described earlier. Inagaki et al. (2016) showed *greater* ventral striatum response in lonely participants when seeing images of close others (vs. strangers) compared with non-lonely individuals, and D'Agostino et al. (2019) found *no* significant differences in subjects' ventral striatum response when looking at pleasant and unpleasant social and non-social images. These mixed results may be due to differences in sample characteristics and exact tasks. Although the ventral striatum response was different, these results are not necessarily inconsistent. D'Agostino and colleagues noted that they used different sets of images with two people interacting, as opposed to the images of one or two non-interacting people that had been used by Cacioppo and colleagues. Additionally, lonely individuals could have diminished ventral striatum activation in response to pleasant social images but still possibly crave social interactions and have increased activation when shown pictures of close others. Lastly, each of the studies had different samples; notably, D'Agostino and colleagues included two discrete age ranges of younger (18–28 years) and older (55–88 years) individuals, whereas the other two studies only included younger adults, and one of these two used a small, all-female sample (Bocincova et al. 2019). There may be different activation patterns with aging, although the chronicity of loneliness is likely to be a factor as well as emotional versus social loneliness and individual differences.

Overall, lonely individuals appear to have differential reactions to negative stimuli, especially in the reward circuitry regions of the brain. Although some of the evidence is mixed, lonely individuals have a different reward region response to social stimuli, indicating that loneliness may be associated with altered social approach motivation. Research derived from socially isolated rodent models and social rejection experiments in humans demonstrates that social approach motivation increases after social isolation due to dopaminergic activity (see Cacioppo et al. 2014 for review). The relationship between loneliness and social drive among humans is less clear; studies seem to suggest that loneliness is associated with decreased socialization motivation. Although this may seem counterintuitive, from an evolutionary perspective, lonely individuals may have had to be hypervigilant and distrustful of others to boost reproductive viability. The causality of the underlying correlation between loneliness and decreased social motivation remains unclear.

Another area of study in task-based fMRI addresses loneliness-related differences in brain activation during self- and social reflection tasks. Courtney and Meyer (2020) found that loneliness is associated with changes in neural representations of self in relation to others in the medial PFC (mPFC) and posterior cingulate cortex during a reflection task. Golde et al. (2019) found that loneliness in adolescents was related to lower ventromedial PFC (vmPFC) activation during self-referential processing. Collectively, these results indicate that the mPFC may play a role in self-referential processing and activate differentially in lonely individuals than in non-lonely individuals when they are thinking about self or others.

Lastly, task-based fMRI studies have examined the effects of loneliness in psychiatric populations. One study examined a sample of patients with schizophrenia and found that individuals with increased loneliness were more likely to have insula activation to expressions of disgust (Lindner et al. 2014) and that this activation was positively correlated with loneliness. This suggests that people with schizophrenia who are lonely may be more primed for negative facial expressions given that the insula is a region known to be involved in emotions, including fear. Another study examining older individuals with late-life depression found that loneliness was related to connectivity differences in the subcortical regions of the salience network (including the amygdala) (Wong et al. 2016). Lastly, one study examined how adults with depression and loneliness responded to a working memory task. The authors found that loneliness was positively associated with inferior parietal cortex–rostral dmPFC connectivity. Because the mPFC is associated with self-referential processing, the authors suggested that lonely individuals show increased regulation of this process, which could be related to the fact that loneliness is associated with negative social cognitive biases. This study also gives secondary evidence that loneliness is linked to changes in cognitive processes (Gao et al. 2020).

Despite the advantages of fMRI, current research findings are limited by the heterogeneity of tasks and the lack of replication of these findings. Moreover, the external validity is uncertain because these tasks infer how lonely individuals react in social situations, even though the tasks may involve looking at images or words. In many of these studies, participants passively view tasks in lieu of more direct assessments of motivation, such as willingness to expend effort. Together, these task-based fMRI studies show that loneliness is associated with altered activation of reward circuits and that the PFC may be involved in loneliness.

Electroencephalography

Electroencephalography is another methodology that can be used to understand how lonely brains interact differently than non-lonely brains in different experimental paradigms with greater temporal resolution than fMRIs. A recent review identified three studies that used electroencephalography to examine high-density event-related potentials during different tasks (Bocincova et al. 2019; Cacioppo et al. 2015, 2016). Cacioppo et al. (2015) examined the differences between lonely and non-lonely individuals in temporal response to positive and negative social stimuli in an electroencephalographic task. The results of this study showed that lonely brain microstates differentiated negative social stimuli from negative non-social stimuli faster than non-lonely brains. Another report by the same group of authors had similar findings. In this second publication, loneliness was associated with quicker differentiation of socially threatening images when compared with non-socially threatening images in lonely versus non-lonely individuals (Cacioppo et al. 2016). The authors noted that these findings may be consistent with increased threat surveillance in lonely individuals (Cacioppo and Cacioppo 2018).

Neurocircuitry

Resting-state fMRI scanning is a method of fMRI used to understand how the brain operates when it is not engaged in a task. Many of these studies were exploratory and tried to understand how the brains of lonely individuals were different from with non-lonely brains in a resting-state mode. Some of these studies examined differences in functional resting-state connectivity between regions, whereas others examined differences in functional resting-state connectivity between brain networks.

Two studies linked loneliness with differences in the default mode network (DMN). In a study with 74 patients with major depressive disorder, the authors found that a higher social dysfunction score, which included loneliness, was associated with decreased DMN connectivity, specifically within the mPFC at resting state (Saris et al. 2020). However, a more recent and robust study with about 40,000 individuals in the U.K. Brain Bank sample found different results (Spreng et al. 2020). The authors found that the statistically strongest functional connectivity deviations related to loneliness were in the DMN and gave evidence that loneliness was associated with increased internetwork DMN connectivity.

Other resting-state fMRI studies found associations between loneliness and the attentional and visual networks. One of the first studies examining differences in resting-state connectivity found that loneliness was associated with increased brain-wide functional connectivity in the right central operculum and right supramarginal gyrus while controlling for other psychosocial factors (Layden et al. 2017). After further analyses, the authors inferred that loneliness was associated with increased functional connectivity of several key nodes of the cingulo-opercular attentional network.

Another study also examined the relationship between brain networks and the causal flow between these networks (Tian et al. 2017). The researchers found that lonely individuals had a weaker causal flow from the visual to attentional and affective networks and weaker causal flow between the dorsal attentional network and the ventral attentional network. Given that loneliness was correlated with attentional and visual network differences in both studies (Layden et al. 2017; Tian et al. 2017), the authors hypothesized that these results may be consistent with previous theories about hypervigilance to social cues in lonely individuals.

There is growing evidence that loneliness changes neurocircuitry. A handful of publications have already shown that loneliness is associated with differences in functional connectivity of different regions and differences in default mode, attentional, and visual networks of the brain. Although these results show evidence of the differential circuitry of lonely individuals, they should be cautiously interpreted because the field of resting-state fMRI is in its nascency, and most of these results have yet to be replicated given the vast differences in statistical analysis and methodologies.

Other Methodologies

Other studies have tried to identify neurobiological correlates of loneliness using other methods. Two studies analyzed RNA expression of postmortem brain tissue (Canli et al. 2017, 2018), two used PET to analyze amyloid and tau proteins (d'Oleire Uquillas et al. 2018; Donovan et al. 2016), and one longitudinal cohort study examined the association between postmortem brain tissue and Alzheimer's pathology (Wilson et al. 2007).

Canli et al. (2017, 2018) published two studies of RNA expression and analyzed postmortem brain tissue in the nucleus accumbens and dlPFC, respectively. The investigators identified hundreds of differentially expressed transcripts and genes among lonely compared with non-lonely individuals. Both studies identified a significant association between loneliness and genes associated with Alzheimer's disease (AD). The relationships between loneliness and white matter structures in the brain measures were significantly different between brain-derived neurotrophic factor genotypes, suggesting that genes may impact brain structure and architecture (Meng et al. 2017).

Three studies examined the relationship of loneliness to the risk of AD. Two studies by the same investigators using PET imaging found a significant relationship between loneliness and brain AD biomarkers (d'Oleire Uquillas et al. 2018; Donovan et al. 2016). The investigators found higher amyloid burden, especially in apolipoprotein E ε4 carriers (Donovan et al. 2016), and they also found greater tau pathology in the right entorhinal cortex in an a priori region-of-interest analysis and in the right fusiform gyrus in an exploratory whole-brain analysis (d'Oleire Uquillas et al. 2018). One cohort study of 823 older adults from the Rush Memory and Aging Project found that the risk of developing AD and cognitive decline was significantly higher in lonely compared with non-lonely individuals; however, global AD pathology (β-amyloid plaques, neurofibrillary tangles, or cerebral infarction) in the postmortem brains analyzed ($N=90$) showed no significant relationship to loneliness (Wilson et al. 2007), in contrast to the PET studies. In their prospective longitudinal white matter study, Duan et al. (2017) demonstrated that increases in loneliness were correlated to decreases in cognitive function scores and increases in white matter hyperintensities, which are associated with an increased risk of cognitive impairment and dementia.

Overall, these findings align with growing meta-analytic evidence that loneliness is positively associated with an increased risk of dementia (Lara et al. 2019). Loneliness and dementia have strong overlap in genetics, be-

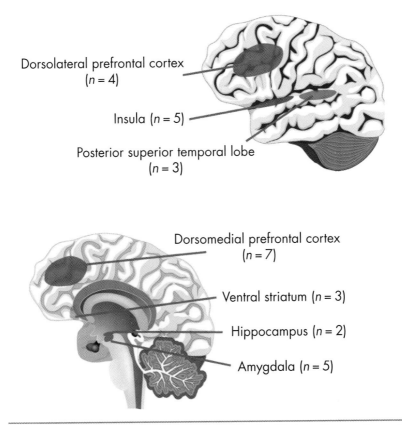

Dorsolateral prefrontal cortex
(*n* = 4)

Insula (*n* = 5)

Posterior superior temporal lobe
(*n* = 3)

Dorsomedial prefrontal cortex
(*n* = 7)

Ventral striatum (*n* = 3)

Hippocampus (*n* = 2)

Amygdala (*n* = 5)

FIGURE 6–1. **Brain regions associated with loneliness, based on published findings.**

Source. Adapted from Lam et al. 2021.

havioral symptoms, physical health risk factors, and stress/inflammatory responses (Hawkley and Cacioppo 2010). The current literature strongly suggests that loneliness is related to AD.

Neurobiology of Loneliness

Brain Regions Associated With Loneliness

Based on current literature, loneliness appears to be most linked to structural and functional differences in the PFC, insula, hippocampus, amygdala, and posterior superior temporal cortex (pSTC) (Figure 6–1).

The PFC, most notably the mPFC and dlPFC, is strongly associated with loneliness. It was associated with loneliness in most of the studies examined in a recent review, with significant differences found in structure or functional components (activation with social vs. non-social images and functional connectivity) between lonely and non-lonely brains. The PFC is responsible for higher-order executive functions such as focusing attention, emotional regulation, and impulse control. Evolutionarily, the PFC was one of the last structures of the brain to develop. Although PFC subdivisions are not universally agreed upon, the mPFC is generally medial of the lateral PFC and can be further divided into the dmPFC and vmPFC (see Carlén 2017 for anatomical image review). The dlPFC is a part of the PFC that is implicated in working memory, executive functioning, and emotional processing. The mPFC is implicated in self-referential processes (i.e., how one sees oneself), such as self-criticism and social situations. The strong link between the PFC and loneliness is consistent with loneliness being a complex socioemotional trait. The current literature indicates a strong link between the PFC and loneliness, although directionality and causality have yet to be determined.

There is modest evidence that the insula is associated with loneliness. The insula somatic marker hypothesis states that the insula receives and integrates information to create a "global emotional moment." The anterior insula plays a role in various behaviors including emotions, pain, and self-awareness. The insula was reportedly associated with loneliness in studies of gray matter, white matter connectivity, and task-based activation. Evidence indicates that social rejection activates the bilateral anterior insula, which are the same regions activated by physical pain, although some of these findings are mixed. Collectively, these results indicate that loneliness may be associated with differential insular activation to social stimuli, notably negative social stimuli. They are consistent with previous evolutionary theories of loneliness predicting that loneliness leads to increased hypervigilance and sensitivity to rejection (Cacioppo and Cacioppo 2018).

There is moderate evidence that the ventral striatum and other reward structures are associated with loneliness, although some of the findings are not consistent. The ventral striatum, which includes the nucleus accumbens, plays a crucial role in the reinforcement of rewards. Two studies of the reward regions indicated lower activation in lonely individuals (Cacioppo and Hawkley 2009; Tomova et al. 2020), whereas two others had nonsignificant or increased activation (D'Agostino et al. 2019; Inagaki et al. 2016). Research on social isolation in animal models indicates that isolation may change individuals' motivation to approach others. Although some of the results are mixed, the experimental paradigms were different, and further studies will need to confirm how loneliness affects social approach motivation. Overall, there is evidence that loneliness alters the ventral striatum and the reward pathway.

There is mixed evidence that the amygdala is linked to loneliness. The amygdala is a part of the limbic system and is implicated in fear and emotional processing. Most of the studies found an association between gray matter volume or task-based activation in lonely individuals, although one fMRI study found no relationship between loneliness and the amygdala. Given that loneliness is associated with increased rejection sensitivity and attunement to negative social cues, the relationship between the amygdala and loneliness seems consistent.

The link between the pSTC, hippocampus, and cerebellum and loneliness is less clear. Some studies have identified these regions as associated with loneliness, but further confirmatory evidence is needed. The pSTC is implicated in social cognition, including perception of language, speech, and other social signals. Studies have found an association between loneliness and pSTC gray or white matter. The hippocampus is best known for its role in memory. Multiple studies have found a link between loneliness and hippocampal gray matter volume, white matter volume, and functional activity during a social exclusion task. The findings of hippocampal differences in lonely individuals could be due to increased stress and stress-related hormones, such as cortisol. Alternatively, higher loneliness could result in reduced social engagement, leading to hippocampal atrophy. The main function of the cerebellum is sensorimotor coordination, but some evidence also implicates this structure in cognitive and affective processes. Three studies found an association of loneliness with cerebellar gray matter volume, white matter structural efficiency, and connectivity with the visual cortex; however, different subregions of the cerebellum were involved in different reports, indicating uncertainty about its specific role in loneliness.

Brain Networks Associated With Loneliness

Newer research from large neuroimaging and behavioral studies has found associations between loneliness and differences in the function of the default mode, attentional, and visual networks.

The DMN and regions associated with it have been found to be associated with loneliness in numerous studies, including one well-designed study involving more than 40,000 participants. The DMN is a network in the brain known to be active when individuals are not engaged in any other tasks or are engaged in internally focused tasks and is linked with rumination, low mood states, and mental representations of self and others across time and space. The DMN consists of the mPFC, posterior cingulate cortex/precuneus, and angular gyrus. Given the strong association between the DMN and loneliness, some authors hypothesize that this reflects increased mental representation of imagined or desired social interactions.

There is also evidence that loneliness is associated with differences in the attentional and visual networks and the structures associated with these networks in the human brain. The attentional system is the part of the brain responsible for filtering relevant and irrelevant information and is made up of multiple circuits with anatomically distinct borders. Visual systems are responsible for processing and interpreting visual stimuli. Both networks are involved in interpreting and filtering stimuli, especially social stimuli; thus, some hypothesize that loneliness is associated with an altered amount of attention paid to social cues and possible hyperawareness of these cues, which may have provided an evolutionary advantage for lonely individuals. Table 6–1 provides a summary of the selected literature on the neurobiology of loneliness.

Summary

This chapter gives evidence that loneliness is associated with the PFC, insula, and ventral striatum brain structures and with the default mode, attentional, and visual networks. Together, there is strong evidence that loneliness is associated with differences in social brain regions, including the parts responsible for mental representations of self and the affective, perceptual, and attentional systems. Loneliness also has a strong relationship with dementia, specifically AD. These results demonstrate clear evidence that specific brain structures, functionality, and pathology changes are associated with the experience of loneliness. Investigators will need to continue to replicate and expand the quantity and quality of the studies to understand the specific neurobiological mechanisms underlying loneliness. Collectively, the current literature gives evidence that loneliness may increase hypervigilance and alter social approach motivation, which supports the theory that loneliness evolved as a means to increase reproductive fitness.

KEY POINTS

- Individuals who are lonely show changes in brain structure and functioning across a variety of neurobiological assessments.

- Neurobiological changes in loneliness consistently highlight brain regions that are essential for social cognition.

- Future studies should examine the impact of loneliness interventions on brain function to better understand the underlying mechanisms of social functioning.

TABLE 6–1. Selective publications by brain region and network

Structure—Proposed function	Study	Study summary	Findings
PFC—Behavioral regulation, attentional and inhibitory control, and response selection	Ehlers et al. 2017	Longitudinal, 247 older adults	Larger PFC baseline volume moderated decreases in loneliness over course of intervention.
	Cristofori et al. 2019	Cohort, 132 veterans with TBI (11 right PFC lesions)	Lesions in right PFC resulted in lower loneliness in patients with TBI.
mPFC—Self-referential processing, such as self-referential criticism in social situations; also involved in mesolimbic dopamine pathway; also considered part of the DMN	Eisenberger et al. 2007	Task-based fMRI, 30 healthy young adults	Greater left mPFC response when completing Cyberball task associated with loneliness.
	Cacioppo et al. 2009	Task-based fMRI, 23 healthy young adults	Lower dmPFC response when looking at pleasant social images and higher dmPFC response when looking at pleasant non-social images associated with loneliness.
	Nakagawa et al. 2015	White matter, 776 healthy young adults	Lower left dmPFC regional white matter density associated with loneliness.
	Golde et al. 2019	Task-based fMRI, 41 adolescents	Lower vmPFC activation during self-processing task associated with loneliness among adolescents.
	Courtney and Meyer 2020	Task-based fMRI, 43 college students	Less similarity in self-/other neural representation in mPFC among lonely individuals, possibly representing a lonelier "neural self" consistent with the idea that lonely individuals may feel more distant from others.

TABLE 6–1. Selective publications by brain region and network *(continued)*

Structure—Proposed function	Study	Study summary	Findings
mPFC—Self-referential processing *(continued)*	Gao et al. 2020	Task-based fMRI, 44 middle-aged adults (depression vs. healthy control subjects)	Functional connectivity between the rostral dmPFC cortex and inferior parietal cortex positively associated with loneliness during working memory task.
	Kiesow et al. 2020	Gray matter, 10,129 individuals	Greater amygdala volumetric differences among lonely and non-lonely females compared with males.
dlPFC—Working memory, executive functioning, emotional processing, cognitive empathy	Düzel et al. 2019	Gray matter, 319 healthy older adults	Loneliness associated with lower dlPFC gray matter volume. Significant loneliness by age interaction: older adults reporting a higher level of perceived loneliness linked to lower volumes in dlPFC. In contrast, younger older adults reporting higher loneliness showed higher volumes in dlPFC. Significant loneliness-by-depression interaction: lonely individuals with depression had even lower gray matter volume in dlPFC.
	Feng et al. 2019	Resting state fMRI, 75 healthy young adults	dlPFC is key node that contributed to resting-fMRI predictive model of loneliness.
	Kong et al. 2015	Gray matter, 308 healthy young adults	Increased dlPFC gray volume associated with loneliness.
	Liu et al. 2016	Gray matter, 405 healthy young adults	dlPFC GMV's association with attitudes toward suicide was mediated by loneliness.

TABLE 6–1. Selective publications by brain region and network *(continued)*

Structure—Proposed function	Study	Study summary	Findings
Insula—Integration of sensory, interoceptive, and emotional information	Lindner et al. 2014	Task-based fMRI, 76 patients (patients with schizophrenia vs. healthy control subjects)	Higher bilateral insula activation in response to disgust associated with loneliness in individuals with schizophrenia.
Anterior insula—Empathy for pain	Cacioppo et al. 2009	Task-based fMRI, 23 healthy young adults	Higher left anterior insula activation when looking at pleasant social vs. pleasant non-social images; difference associated with loneliness.
	Tian et al. 2014	White matter, 30 healthy young adults	Poorer connectivity of white matter tracts of anterior insula to other nodes of ventral attentional network associated with loneliness.
	Nakagawa et al. 2015	White matter, 776 healthy young adults	Lower right anterior insula regional white matter density associated with loneliness.
	Cristofori et al. 2019	Longitudinal, 132 veterans with TBI (28 right anterior insula lesions)	Lesions in anterior insula resulted in decreased loneliness in patients with TBI.
	Düzel et al. 2019	Gray matter, 319 healthy older adults	Lower insula GMV associated with loneliness. Significant loneliness-by depression interaction: lonely individuals with depression had even lower GMV in insula.

TABLE 6–1. Selective publications by brain region and network *(continued)*

Structure—Proposed function	Study	Study summary	Findings
Amygdala—Fear processing	Tian et al. 2016	Gray matter, 118 healthy young adults	Positive association between left amygdala volume and social distress score mediated by loneliness.
	Wong et al. 2016	Task-based fMRI, 54 older adults (patients with late-life depression vs. healthy control subjects)	Weaker amygdala to superior frontal gyrus connectivity associated with loneliness.
	Ehlers et al. 2017	Longitudinal, 247 older adults	Amygdala GMV associated with loneliness. Larger baseline amygdala volumes associated with greater decreases in loneliness over course of intervention.
	Düzel et al. 2019	Gray matter, 319 healthy older adults	Less GMV in left amygdala/anterior hippocampus and left posterior parahippocampus associated with loneliness. Significant loneliness-by-age interaction for amygdala and hippocampus: older adults reporting a higher level of perceived loneliness linked to lower volumes in hippocampus and higher volume in amygdala compared with younger adults with high levels of loneliness.
	Kiesow et al. 2020	Gray matter, 10,129 individuals	Greater amygdala volumetric differences among lonely and non-lonely males compared with females.

TABLE 6–1. Selective publications by brain region and network *(continued)*

Structure—Proposed function	Study	Study summary	Findings
Structures associated with reward pathway—Reward reinforcement	Cacioppo et al. 2009	Task-based fMRI, 23 healthy young adults	Lower VS response when looking at pleasant social images and higher VS response when looking at pleasant non-social images associated with loneliness.
	Inagaki et al. 2016	Task-based fMRI	Greater activation of VS when seeing images of close others (compared to strangers) associated with loneliness.
	Sin et al. 2018	Gray matter, 52 older adults (patients with multiple episodes of depression *vs.* single episode *vs.* healthy control subjects)	VS GMV affected by recurrence of depressive episodes.
	Tomova et al. 2020	Task-based fMRI, 40 adults	Fasting from food or social connection similarly activated SN/VTA. Loneliness associated with decreased activation in SN/VTA compared with non-lonely individuals.
Superior temporal lobe—Perception of language, speech, and other social signals, such as biological motion and gaze direction	Cacioppo et al. 2009	Task-based fMRI, 23 healthy young adults	Higher bilateral superior temporal gyrus activation when looking at unpleasant social *vs.* unpleasant non-social images; difference associated with loneliness.
	Kanai et al. 2012	Gray matter, 108 healthy young adults	Lower pSTS GMV associated with loneliness.
	Nakagawa et al. 2015	White matter, 776 healthy young adults	Lower left pSTS regional white matter density associated with loneliness.

TABLE 6–1. Selective publications by brain region and network *(continued)*

Structure—Proposed function	Study	Study summary	Findings
Hippocampus—Memory encoding	Eisenberger et al. 2007	Task-based fMRI, 30 healthy young adults	Greater left hippocampus response when completing Cyberball task associated with loneliness.
	Düzel et al. 2019	Gray matter, 319 healthy older adults	Less GMV in left amygdala/anterior hippocampus and left posterior parahippocampus associated with loneliness. Significant loneliness-by-age interaction for amygdala and hippocampus: older adults reporting a higher level of perceived loneliness linked to lower volumes in hippocampus compared with younger adults with high levels of loneliness.
Cerebellum—Sensorimotor coordination and affective processes	Düzel et al. 2019	Gray matter, 319 healthy older adults	Less GMV in left cerebellum associated with loneliness.
	Wong et al. 2019	Gray matter/task-based fMRI, 99 all-ages adults	Multiple regions of cerebellum (vermis Lobule VI and vermis crus II) differed among those who were susceptible and non-susceptible to loneliness. Greater posterior cerebellum functional connectivity to right visual cortex when presented positive words in task-based fMRI associated with loneliness.
Visual systems	Cacioppo et al. 2009	Task-based fMRI, 23 healthy young adults	Higher bilateral visual cortex activation when looking at unpleasant social vs. unpleasant non-social images; difference associated with loneliness.

TABLE 6–1. Selective publications by brain region and network (*continued*)

Structure—Proposed function	Study	Study summary	Findings
Visual systems (*continued*)	Tian et al. 2016	Resting-state fMRI, 30 healthy young adults	Decreased causal flow from affective to visual network in individuals with high loneliness score.
	Mwilambwe-Tshilobo et al. 2019	Resting-state fMRI, 942 healthy older adults	Lower modularity or increased integration between visual brain regions and default and frontoparietal networks in individuals with high loneliness scores.
	Kiesow et al. 2020	Gray matter, 10,129 individuals	Volume of visual sensory network (composed of fusiform gyrus, pSTS, and middle temporal V5 area) deviated between lonely and non-lonely women but not in men.
Attentional network—Orienting and executive control	Tian et al. 2014	White matter, 30 healthy young adults	Poorer connectivity of white matter tracts that linked nodes of ventral attentional network associated with loneliness.
	Tian et al. 2016	Resting-state fMRI, 30 healthy young adults	Decreased causal flow from dorsal attentional network to ventral attentional network flow associated with loneliness.
	Layden et al. 2017	Resting-state fMRI, 55 young healthy adults	Increased functional connectivity in brain regions associated with cingulo-opercular network associated with loneliness.

TABLE 6–1. Selective publications by brain region and network (*continued*)

Structure—Proposed function	Study	Study summary	Findings
DMN—Activates when person is not focused on outside world and when person is daydreaming or mind-wandering	Wong et al. 2016	Task-based fMRI, 54 older adults (patients with late-life depression vs. healthy control subjects)	Increased functional connectivity within DMN associated with loneliness among individuals with late-life depression but decreased functional connectivity in healthy control subjects.
	Saris et al. 2020	Resting-state fMRI, 74 patients with MDD	Decreased connectivity of DMN, especially within mPFC among MDD patients associated with more loneliness and social dysfunction.
	Spreng et al. 2020	Gray matter, white matter, resting-state fMRI, 38,701 from U.K. Biobank	Loneliness associated with increased GMV, white matter microstructural integrity, and stronger functional communication in regions associated with DMN.

Note. dlPFC=dorsolateral prefrontal cortex; DMN=default mode network; dmPFC=dorsomedial prefrontal cortex; fMRI=functional MRI; GMV=gray matter volume; MDD=major depressive disorder; mPFC=medial prefrontal cortex; PFC=prefrontal cortex; pSTS=posterior superior temporal sulcus; SN/ VTA= substantia nigra/ventral tegmental area; TBI=traumatic brain injury; VS=ventral striatum; vmPFC=ventromedial prefrontal cortex.

Source. Adapted from Lam et al. 2021.

Suggested Readings

Cacioppo S, Capitanio JP, Cacioppo JT: Toward a neurology of loneliness. Psychol Bull 140(6):1464–1504, 2014 25222636

Cacioppo JT, Cacioppo S: Loneliness in the modern age: an evolutionary theory of loneliness (ETL). Adv Exp Soc Psychol 58:127–197, 2018

Lam JA, Murray ER, Yu KE, et al: Neurobiology of loneliness: a systematic review. Neuropsychopharmacology 46(11):1873–1887, 2021 34230607

Zovetti N, Rossetti MG, Perlini C, et al: Neuroimaging studies exploring the neural basis of social isolation. Epidemiol Psychiatr Sci 30:e29, 2021 33820592

References

Abdellaoui A, Sanchez-Roige S, Sealock J, et al: Phenome-wide investigation of health outcomes associated with genetic predisposition to loneliness. Hum Mol Genet 28(22):3853–3865, 2019 31518406

Barbey AK, Koenigs M, Grafman J: Dorsolateral prefrontal contributions to human working memory. Cortex 49(5):1195–1205, 2013 22789779

Beutel ME, Klein EM, Brähler E, et al: Loneliness in the general population: prevalence, determinants and relations to mental health. BMC Psychiatry 17(1):97, 2017 28320380

Bocincova A, Nelson T, Johnson J, Routledge C: Experimentally induced nostalgia reduces the amplitude of the event-related negativity. Soc Neurosci 14(6):631–634, 2019 30747030

Brown EG, Gallagher S, Creaven AM: Loneliness and acute stress reactivity: a systematic review of psychophysiological studies. Psychophysiology 55(5):e13031, 2018 29152761

Cacioppo JT, Cacioppo S: Loneliness in the modern age: an evolutionary theory of loneliness (ETL). Adv Exp Soc Psychol 58:127–197, 2018

Cacioppo JT, Hawkley LC: Perceived social isolation and cognition. Trends Cogn Sci 13:447–454, 2009

Cacioppo JT, Norris CJ, Decety J, et al: In the eye of the beholder: individual differences in perceived social isolation predict regional brain activation to social stimuli. J Cogn Neurosci 21(1):83–92, 2009 18476760

Cacioppo JT, Cacioppo S, Boomsma DI: Evolutionary mechanisms for loneliness. Cogn Emotion 28(1):3–21, 2014 24067110

Cacioppo S, Balogh S, Cacioppo JT: Implicit attention to negative social, in contrast to nonsocial, words in the Stroop task differs between individuals high and low in loneliness: evidence from event-related brain microstates. Cortex 70:213–233, 2015 26195152

Cacioppo S, Bangee M, Balogh S, et al: Loneliness and implicit attention to social threat: a high-performance electrical neuroimaging study. Cogn Neurosci 7(1-4):138–159, 2016 26274315

Canli T, Wen R, Wang X, et al: Differential transcriptome expression in human nucleus accumbens as a function of loneliness. Mol Psychiatry 22(7):1069–1078, 2017 27801889

Canli T, Yu L, Yu X, et al: Loneliness 5 years ante-mortem is associated with disease-related differential gene expression in postmortem dorsolateral prefrontal cortex. Transl Psychiatry 8(1):2, 2018 29317593

Carlén M: What constitutes the prefrontal cortex? Science 358(6362):478–482, 2017 29074767

Courtney AL, Meyer ML: Self-other representation in the social brain reflects social connection. J Neurosci 40(29):5616–5627, 2020 32541067

Cristofori I, Pal S, Zhong W, et al: The lonely brain: evidence from studying patients with penetrating brain injury. Soc Neurosci 14(6):663–675, 2019 30501456

D'Agostino AEK, Kattan D, Canli T: An fMRI study of loneliness in younger and older adults. Soc Neurosci 14(2):136–148, 2019 29471719

d'Oleire Uquillas F, Jacobs HIL, Biddle KD, et al: Regional tau pathology and loneliness in cognitively normal older adults. Transl Psychiatry 8(1):282, 2018 30563962

Donovan NJ, Okereke OI, Vannini P, et al: Association of higher cortical amyloid burden with loneliness in cognitively normal older adults. JAMA Psychiatry 73(12):1230–1237, 2016 27806159

Duan D, Dong Y, Zhang H, et al: Empty-nest-related psychological distress is associated with progression of brain white matter lesions and cognitive impairment in the elderly. Sci Rep 7:43816, 2017 28256594

Düzel S, Drewelies J, Gerstorf D, et al: Structural brain correlates of loneliness among older adults. Sci Rep 9(1):13569, 2019 31537846

Ehlers DK, Daugherty AM, Burzynska AZ, et al: Regional brain volumes moderate, but do not mediate, the effects of group-based exercise training on reductions in loneliness in older adults. Front Aging Neurosci 9:110, 2017 28487648

Eisenberger NI, Gable SL, Lieberman MD: Functional magnetic resonance imaging responses relate to differences in real-world social experience. Emotion 7:745–754, 2007

Feng C, Wang L, Li T, Xu P: Connectome-based individualized prediction of loneliness. Soc Cogn Affect Neurosci 14:353–365, 2019

Gao J, Davis LK, Hart AB, et al: Genome-wide association study of loneliness demonstrates a role for common variation. Neuropsychopharmacology 42(4):811–821, 2017 27629369

Gao M, Shao R, Huang CM, et al: The relationship between loneliness and working-memory-related frontoparietal network connectivity in people with major depressive disorder. Behav Brain Res 393:112776, 2020 32615139

Golde S, Romund L, Lorenz RC, et al: Loneliness and adolescents' neural processing of self, friends, and teachers: consequences for the school self-concept. J Res Adolesc 29(4):938–952, 2019 30019816

Hawkley LC, Cacioppo JT: Loneliness matters: a theoretical and empirical review of consequences and mechanisms. Ann Behav Med 40(2):218–227, 2010 20652462

Holt-Lunstad J, Smith TB, Baker M, et al: Loneliness and social isolation as risk factors for mortality: a meta-analytic review. Perspect Psychol Sci 10(2):227–237, 2015 25910392

Inagaki TKM, Muscatell KA, Moieni M, et al: Yearning for connection? Loneliness is associated with increased ventral striatum activity to close others. Soc Cogn Affect Neurosci 11(7):1096–1101, 2016 26084531

Kanai R, Bahrami B, Duchaine B, et al: Brain structure links loneliness to social perception. Curr Biol 22(20):1975–1979, 2012 23041193

Kiesow H, Dunbar RI, Kable JW, et al: 10,000 social brains: sex differentiation in human brain anatomy. Science Advances 6(12):eaaz1170, 2020

Klinenberg E: Is loneliness a health epidemic? New York Times, February 9, 2018, p SR8

Kong X, Wei D, Li W, et al: Neuroticism and extraversion mediate the association between loneliness and the dorsolateral prefrontal cortex. Exp Brain Res 233:157–164, 2015

Kuiper JS, Zuidersma M, Oude Voshaar RC, et al: Social relationships and risk of dementia: a systematic review and meta-analysis of longitudinal cohort studies. Ageing Res Rev 22:39–57, 2015 25956016

Lam JA, Murray ER, Yu KE, et al: Neurobiology of loneliness: a systematic review. Neuropsychopharmacology 46(11):1873–1887, 2021 34230607

Lara E, Martín-María N, De la Torre-Luque A, et al: Does loneliness contribute to mild cognitive impairment and dementia? A systematic review and meta-analysis of longitudinal studies. Ageing Res Rev 52:7–16, 2019 30914351

Layden EA, Cacioppo JT, Cacioppo S, et al: Perceived social isolation is associated with altered functional connectivity in neural networks associated with tonic alertness and executive control. Neuroimage 145:58–73, 2017

Lindner C, Dannlowski U, Walhöfer K, et al: Social alienation in schizophrenia patients: association with insula responsiveness to facial expressions of disgust. PLoS One 9(1):e85014, 2014 24465469

Liu H, Wang Y, Liu W, et al: Neuroanatomical correlates of attitudes toward suicide in a large healthy sample: a voxel-based morphometric analysis. Neuropsychologia 80:185–193, 2016

Meng J, Hao L, Wei D, et al: BDNF Val66Met polymorphism modulates the effect of loneliness on white matter microstructure in young adults. Biol Psychol 130:41–49, 2017 28988974

Mwilambwe-Tshilobo L, Ge T, Chong M, et al: Loneliness and meaning in life are reflected in the intrinsic network architecture of the brain. Soc Cogn Affect Neurosci 14:423–433, 2019

Nakagawa S, Takeuchi H, Taki Y, et al: White matter structures associated with loneliness in young adults. Sci Rep 5:17001, 2015

National Academies of Sciences, Engineering, and Medicine: Social Isolation and Loneliness in Older Adults: Opportunities for the Health Care System. Washington, DC, The National Academies Press, 2020

Rico-Uribe LA, Caballero FF, Martín-María N, et al: Association of loneliness with all-cause mortality: a meta-analysis. PLoS One 13(1):e0190033, 2018 29300743

Saris IMJ, Penninx BWJH, Dinga R, et al: Default mode network connectivity and social dysfunction in major depressive disorder. Sci Rep 10(1):194, 2020 31932627

Sin ELL, Liu HL, Lee SH, et al: The relationships between brain structural changes and perceived loneliness in older adults suffering from late-life depression. Int J Geriatr Psychiatry 33:606–612, 2018

Smith KJ, Gavey S, RIddell NE, et al: The association between loneliness, social isolation and inflammation: a systematic review and meta-analysis. Neurosci Biobehav Rev 112:519–541, 2020 32092313

Spreng RN, Dimas E, Mwilambwe-Tshilobo L, et al: The default network of the human brain is associated with perceived social isolation. Nat Commun 11(1):6393, 2020 33319780

Steptoe A, Shankar A, Demakakos P, Wardle J: Social isolation, loneliness, and all-cause mortality in older men and women. Proc Natl Acad Sci USA 110(15):5797–5801, 2013 23530191

Tian X, Hou X, Wang K, et al: Neuroanatomical correlates of individual differences in social anxiety in a non-clinical population. Soc Neurosci 11:424–437, 2016

Tian Y, Liang S, Yuan Z, et al: White matter structure in loneliness: preliminary findings from diffusion tensor imaging. Neuroreport 25:843–847, 2014

Tian Y, Yang L, Chen S, et al: Causal interactions in resting-state networks predict perceived loneliness. PloS One 12:e0177443, 2017

Tomova L, Wang KL, Thompson T, et al: Acute social isolation evokes midbrain craving responses similar to hunger. Nat Neurosci 23(12):1597-1605, 2020 33230328

Valtorta NK, Kanaan M, Gilbody S, et al: Loneliness and social isolation as risk factors for coronary heart disease and stroke: systematic review and meta-analysis of longitudinal observational studies. Heart 102(13):1009–1016, 2016 27091846

Wilson RS, Krueger KR, Arnold SE, et al: Loneliness and risk of Alzheimer disease. Arch Gen Psychiatry 64(2):234–240, 2007 17283291

Wong NML, Liu HL, Lin C, et al: Loneliness in late-life depression: structural and functional connectivity during affective processing. Psychol Med 46(12):2485–2499, 2016 27328861

Wong NML, Shao R, Yeung PPS, et al: Negative affect shared with siblings is associated with structural brain network efficiency and loneliness in adolescents. Neuroscience 421:39–47, 2019

7

Systemic Neuroendocrine and Inflammatory Mechanisms in Loneliness

Kelly E. Rentscher, Ph.D.
Steve W. Cole, Ph.D.
Judith E. Carroll, Ph.D.

LONELINESS HAS BEEN associated with increased risk for adverse mental and physical health outcomes, including depression (Cacioppo et al. 2006, 2010), cardiovascular disease and stroke (Holt-Lunstad and Smith 2016), cancer progression (Bower et al. 2018; Lutgendorf and Andersen 2015; Lutgendorf et al. 2020), loss of motor function (Buchman et al. 2010), and cognitive declines (Cacioppo and Hawkley 2009). In addition, a meta-analysis by Holt-Lunstad et al. (2015) found that loneliness was associated with a 26% increased risk of all-cause mortality that is comparable in magnitude to well-established risk factors such as obesity and smoking. This growing literature has led researchers to call for loneliness to be regarded as a public health priority (Holt-Lunstad et al. 2017). However, the biological pathways through which loneliness exerts its health effects are only beginning to be understood. In this chapter, we review one domain of mechanistic research that has helped to clarify how loneliness might increase the risk of multiple chronic diseases through neural and endocrine alterations that stimulate inflammatory biology and thereby accelerate the development and progression of cardiovascular, neurodegenerative, and neoplastic (cancer) diseases.

In their evolutionary theory of loneliness (ETL), Cacioppo and Cacioppo (2018) posited that loneliness is a motivational state that serves an evolutionary function. They outlined that because reliable social relationships can contribute to the likelihood of reproduction and survival, individuals are motivated to maintain beneficial social connections. Similar to the way that aversion to physical pain motivates behaviors to promote survival, an aversion to loneliness serves as a biological warning signal that alerts individuals to a threat to their social system and motivates them to repair important relationships. At the same time, the ETL posits that loneliness can also trigger behaviors such as increased vigilance to threat, avoidance of socially threatening circumstances, and a focus on one's self-interests and protection, as well as biological responses that promote short-term survival. These threat-related physiological changes include activation of peripheral threat defense systems including the sympathetic nervous system (SNS) and hypothalamic-pituitary-adrenal (HPA) axis. As outlined in the ETL, transient activation of these systems during brief periods of isolation has likely been adaptive throughout our evolutionary history to prepare the body for the changing survival challenges associated with the lack of social support (e.g., increased risk of injury due to predation or conspecific violence). However, this connection between lonely experience and threat-responsive physiology implies that prolonged periods of chronic loneliness (which typically characterize about 20% of the population in contemporary societies) essentially induce a state of chronic stress physiology.

Chronic stress has multiple adverse effects across physiological systems, including the immune system (O'Connor et al. 2021; Segerstrom and Miller 2004). In the context of the immune system, Irwin and Cole (2011) provided one model for understanding how neuroendocrine and inflammatory mechanisms ultimately impact general immune system homeostasis, particularly in the context of the innate immune system. When an individual perceives a threat in the environment, the CNS responds by releasing catecholamines (e.g., norepinephrine) from the nerve fibers of the SNS and glucocorticoids (e.g., cortisol) from the HPA axis. Through these neuroeffector molecules, the CNS interacts with receptors on the surface of immune cells (i.e., leukocytes) to regulate the expression of immune response genes, such as those involved in inflammation or antiviral response.

In this model, immune mediators such as inflammatory cytokines can also feed back to regulate CNS function and influence a person's perceptions and behaviors. For instance, the presence of proinflammatory cytokines in the brain can decrease neurotransmitters such as noradrenaline, dopamine, and serotonin (Miller et al. 2009) and interact with interleukin (IL)-1 receptors in the hypothalamus and hippocampus (Dantzer et al. 2008; Hart 1988). Loneliness, as a form of social-ecological threat perceived by the CNS, may therefore influence the immune system through SNS and HPA pathways. This results in an inflammatory response that can further increase perceptions of threat via amygdala activation pathways, prompting social withdrawal and reduced reward from social engagement and thereby amplifying and prolonging loneliness through a reciprocal CNS-immune system feedback mechanism (Cacioppo and Cacioppo 2018; Cole et al. 2015a). This chapter reviews how loneliness affects these neuroendocrine and inflammatory mechanisms to increase risk for adverse health outcomes.

Loneliness and SNS Activity

SNS activity, which involves the release of catecholamines such as norepinephrine, is a vital part of the fight-or-flight response to acute stressors. It increases contraction of the heart and skeletal muscle to prepare the body to respond to a perceived or actual threat. Few studies to date have investigated the effects of loneliness on SNS activity, and those few have yielded mixed findings. In a longitudinal study of older adults, Cole et al. (2015b) found that loneliness was associated with elevated urinary norepinephrine levels consistent with neuronal SNS activity. As part of this study, they also developed an innovative model of loneliness in rhesus macaques that ranked animals as high or low in loneliness based on their rates of spontaneous social interaction and behavioral signs of social threat sensitivity during interactions (Cole et al. 2015a). Consistent with the findings in humans, adult male macaques that exhibited higher behavioral indicators of loneliness had elevated urinary norepinephrine levels. In contrast, another study with a population-based sample of adults age 50 years and older did not find an association between perceived loneliness and urinary catecholamine (i.e., epinephrine and norepinephrine) levels from overnight to early morning (Hawkley et al. 2006).

Importantly, SNS nerve fibers also innervate the bone marrow (Elenkov et al. 2000), the soft tissue in bones where most blood cells are formed and differentiate (with the exception of T lymphocytes, which mature in the thymus). It is therefore possible that loneliness, through the release of SNS effector molecules into the bone marrow niche, may also influence the composition of the leukocyte population in circulation. To test this hypothesis, Cole et al. (2015a) used a social threat model in which individually housed male rhesus macaques were randomized to socialize for 5 weeks with either a continuously changing group of novel social partners (chronic social threat) or a stable group of social partners. Relative to the macaques with familiar social partners, those exposed to chronic social threat showed an increase in the proportion of monocytes in circulation—and especially the immature, proinflammatory classical (CD14^{++}/CD16^{-}) subset of monocytes (Cole et al. 2015a). Previous research has demonstrated that, in addition to being inflammation-primed, classical monocytes can themselves traffic to the brain to promote anxiety and alter social behavior (Wohleb et al. 2015) and may therefore also amplify or prolong experiences of loneliness.

Loneliness and HPA Axis Activity

HPA axis activity, which involves the release of glucocorticoids (e.g., cortisol), also plays an important role in the fight-or-flight response to acute stressors because it regulates physiological functions such as metabolism, digestion, and immunity in the face of threat. Cortisol levels typically follow a diurnal pattern in which levels are highest in the morning, lowest in the evening, and peak approximately 30 minutes after awakening, which is referred to as the cortisol awakening response (CAR). Researchers use several metrics to assess cortisol levels, including the CAR, the diurnal slope (calculated from highest to lowest point over the course of a day), the area under the curve (AUC; calculated as total output over the course of a day), and momentary levels in circulation.

Studies that examined the CAR have included a wide age range of participants, typically measured cortisol over 3 consecutive days, and assessed loneliness at the more stable (i.e., trait) and at the daily or momentary (i.e., state) level. In the first study of loneliness-cortisol associations in adolescents, those reporting greater chronic loneliness showed a higher CAR (Zilioli et al. 2017). Several studies with young adults, including first-semester college students, have found that greater daily loneliness was associated with a higher CAR the following morning (Doane and Adam 2010; Pressman et al. 2005; Sladek and Doane 2015), with the exception of one study that collected cortisol for 1 day only (Lai et al. 2018). In a study that compared cortisol levels on weekdays and weekends, women who were high in chronic loneliness showed a higher CAR on weekends than women who were low in loneliness, and no difference between weekdays and weekends, suggesting sustained activation of the HPA axis even on days that are generally considered less stressful (Okamura et al. 2011). Among adults age 50 years and older, greater chronic loneliness has also been associated with a higher CAR (Steptoe et al. 2004); however, studies with older adults have yielded more mixed findings. One found that older adults reporting greater daily loneliness had a higher CAR the following morning (Adam et al. 2006), consistent with findings in younger adults. However, other studies found that older adults and older married men (but not married women) with chronic loneliness showed a lower CAR than those who were not lonely (Johar et al. 2021; Schutter et al. 2017). Interestingly, Schutter et al. (2017) also demonstrated that older adults with chronic loneliness showed a lower suppression of cortisol following dexamethasone (i.e., a synthetic glucocorticoid) administration than those who were not lonely. These latter findings are more consistent with the declines in cortisol levels observed with increasing chronological age and suggest that chronic loneliness may further contribute to these declines.

Although fewer studies have assessed diurnal cortisol slopes, the overall pattern of findings is similar to the CAR studies and more consistent across age groups. In their study of loneliness-cortisol associations in adolescents, Zilioli et al. (2017) also found that those who reported greater loneliness over 3 days showed flatter diurnal cortisol slopes. Studies with young adults have found that greater chronic loneliness was associated with both flatter (Doane and Adam 2010) and steeper (Lai et al. 2018) diurnal slopes; however, the latter only measured cortisol for 1 day. Another study found that among first-semester college students who reported less effective coping during their transition to college, increases in loneliness were associated with flatter diurnal cortisol slopes relative to those with more effective coping (Drake et al. 2016). Consistent with patterns in younger adults, older adults and older married men (but not married women) high in loneliness also had flatter diurnal cortisol slopes than those low in loneliness (Cole et al. 2007; Johar et al. 2021). Overall, studies assessing the relationship of loneliness with cortisol slopes suggest high levels of loneliness are related to flatter diurnal slopes.

To assess total cortisol output over a day, researchers have calculated the AUC and average cortisol levels across the day, yielding mixed findings. One study of undergraduate students found that greater chronic loneliness was associated with a larger AUC (collected for only 1 day; Lai et al. 2018), whereas another study found no association (Pressman et al. 2005). One study found an association between chronic loneliness and average cortisol levels across the day (Cacioppo et al. 2000), but several others did not (Cole et al. 2007; Pressman et al. 2005; Steptoe et al. 2004). One exception is a longitudinal study in which older adults high in loneliness showed a 2-year increase in diurnal cortisol volume; however, the authors noted that the effect was buffered by self-protective coping, suggesting that the association between loneliness and HPA activity might be modifiable (Rueggeberg et al. 2012). Based on the existing literature, total cortisol output appears to be higher among those with greater loneliness.

In addition, a few studies that have assessed momentary levels of cortisol in circulation have found that chronic loneliness was associated with higher urinary cortisol levels in adults who were hospitalized for a psychiatric disorder (Kiecolt-Glaser et al. 1984), but not with urinary or salivary levels in population-based samples (Hawkley et al. 2006; Steptoe et al. 2004). Finally, laboratory-based studies of cortisol reactivity have found that among younger adults with high chronic interpersonal stress, momentary experiences of loneliness were associated with momentary increases in cortisol (Doane and Adam 2010), and women with greater chronic loneliness had a lower cortisol response to an acute stress task (Hackett et al. 2012). These findings suggest that those with higher loneliness may have a more pronounced physiological response to acute stressors, although additional research is needed to disentangle these momentary associations between loneliness, stress, and cortisol.

Researchers have also assessed the sensitivity of glucocorticoid receptors to cortisol signals at the molecular level by measuring patterns of gene expression and corresponding transcription control pathways. Genes are composed of DNA molecules that are transcribed into messenger RNA (mRNA), which then serves as the code for the formation of proteins that carry out functions in the body and can influence behavior (Cole 2014). Transcription factors play an important role in this process because they are proteins that bind to the promoter regions of DNA to regulate (i.e., turn on or off) transcription of the DNA into RNA. In addition to measuring expression levels of target genes (e.g., genes involved in a specific process), the activity of transcription factors can be inferred based on patterns of gene expression that are downstream from a given promoter region (Cole et al. 2005). In a small sample, older adults with chronically high loneliness showed reduced transcription (i.e., underexpression) of genes involved in glucocorticoid receptor signaling (e.g., *HIST1*, *H2BG*, *STAT1*, *TNFRSF17*, *TCN1*) compared to those with low loneliness (Cole et al. 2007). Furthermore, bioinformatics analyses using the Transcript Element Listening System (TELiS; Cole et al. 2005) suggested that older adults with high loneliness also had lower activity (i.e., downregulation) of glucocorticoid receptor transcription factors (i.e., TRANSFAC V$GR_Q6 transcription factor binding motifs) in the promoter regions of overexpressed genes compared to those with low loneliness (Cole et al. 2007). As mentioned earlier, Cole et al. (2015a) behaviorally characterized rhesus macaques as high versus low in loneliness based on rates of spontaneous social interaction and behavioral signs of social threat sensitivity during the interactions. Consistent with findings in humans, rhesus macaques that exhibited higher behavioral indicators of loneliness also showed lower glucocorticoid receptor transcription factor activity in the promoter regions of overexpressed genes relative to animals that exhibited lower indicators of loneliness. Although it did not directly assess transcriptome dynamics related to glucocorticoid receptor sensitivity, another study found that loneliness was associated with reduced leukocyte sensitivity to glucocorticoid regulation (Cole 2008). Specifically, the authors measured the strength of association between cortisol levels and percentage of neutrophils, lymphocytes, and monocytes in circulation and found that older adults who were not lonely demonstrated the expected association between cortisol levels and ratio of neutrophils-to-lymphocytes or neutrophils-to-monocytes in circulation; however, older adults who were lonely did not show an association, suggesting that their leukocytes were not as responsive to the effects of cortisol. Given that glucocorticoids also play a central role in the regulation of inflammation, these findings on glucocorticoid receptor sensitivity are also relevant for understanding associations between loneliness and inflammation (Cole 2008).

Loneliness and Inflammation

Inflammation is an important component of immune system functioning because it is involved in adaptive immune responses that remove pathogens, clear dead or damaged cells from the body, and repair tissue following injury. Researchers use several metrics to assess inflammation, including measuring C-reactive protein (CRP) and proinflammatory cytokine concentrations in plasma as well as measuring the stimulated production of cytokines cells in response to a pathogen (e.g., lipopolysaccharide). Researchers have also assessed inflammatory processes at the molecular level by measuring patterns of gene expression and transcription control pathways.

CRP is an acute-phase protein produced by the liver and a marker of systemic inflammation that is widely used in clinical practice to evaluate cardiovascular and inflammatory diseases. Studies that have investigated associations between loneliness and CRP have yielded mixed findings. For instance, although one population-based study found that adults who were lonely had higher levels of CRP than those who were not (Nersesian et al. 2018), several other studies with middle-aged and older adults did not find an association (Mezuk et al. 2016; O'Luanaigh et al. 2012; Pavela et al. 2018; Shankar et al. 2011; Walker et al. 2019). However, one study found that the onset of loneliness and persistent loneliness over a 4-year period were associated with an increase in CRP over the same period (Vingeliene et al. 2019).

Other key markers of inflammation include cytokines (e.g., IL-6, tumor necrosis factor [TNF]-α) and chemokines (e.g., monocyte chemoattractant protein [MCP]-1), which are proteins produced by leukocytes involved in cell signaling (i.e., cell-to-cell communication) to coordinate the immune response and stimulate the movement of cells to a site of inflammation, infection, or injury. To date, only one study has investigated associations between loneliness and cytokine levels under resting conditions, finding that adults who were lonely had higher IL-6 plasma concentrations than those who were not lonely (Nersesian et al. 2018). Other research has examined loneliness-inflammation associations under conditions of psychological or physiological stress. For instance, young adults with greater sensitivity to social disconnection (which included loneliness) showed higher TNF-α and IL-6 responses to endotoxin, an inflammatory challenge (Moieni et al. 2015). In another study, women with greater loneliness showed larger IL-6 and IL-1 receptor antagonist responses to an acute laboratory stressor and higher MCP-1 levels, but these effects were not observed in men (Hackett et al. 2012). In a study by Jaremka et al. (2013), individuals with higher loneliness who were exposed to an acute laboratory stressor showed greater production of TNF-α and IL-6 in peripheral blood mononuclear cells (PBMCs) stimulated with lipopolysaccharide than individuals who were less lonely. They also found that breast cancer survivors with higher loneliness who were exposed to an acute laboratory stressor showed greater production of IL-6 and IL-1β in PBMCs stimulated with lipopolysaccharide than did those who were less lonely; however, the authors noted that loneliness was not associated with cytokine levels prior to the stressor in both studies. Finally, in a small sample of young men who received either a *Salmonella typhi* vaccination or a placebo, individuals who reported feeling lonelier demonstrated an elevated IL-6 response to the vaccine compared with those who were less lonely (Balter et al. 2019).

As mentioned, researchers have also assessed inflammatory processes by measuring differences in transcriptome dynamics. One pattern of gene expression that several studies have linked to loneliness is the conserved transcriptional response to adversity (CTRA; Cole 2019). The CTRA is characterized by increased transcription (i.e., upregulation) of proinflammatory genes and decreased transcription (i.e., downregulation) of genes involved in type I interferon antiviral responses and immunoglobulin G antibody synthesis in circulating immune cells. The CTRA has been characterized as an evolutionarily adaptive immune response under conditions of social threat (Cole 2019) because individuals who lack companionship may have reduced risk of viral infection from close social interactions and increased risk of microbial threats due to injury or hostile social conditions.

The CTRA pattern was first identified in a sample of older adults, in which individuals with chronically high loneliness showed increased expression of proinflammatory genes (e.g., *EGR3, FOSB, IL1B, IL8, PTGS2*) and decreased expression of antiviral genes (e.g., *STAT1, OAS1, IFI27, IFI6, ISG15*) in circulating immune cells compared with those with low loneliness (Cole et al. 2007). Furthermore, bioinformatics analyses using the TELiS (Cole et al. 2005) suggested that older adults with high chronic loneliness also had a 2.9-fold greater prevalence (i.e., upregulation) of proinflammatory transcription factors (i.e., nuclear factor [NF]-κB/Rel transcription factor binding motifs) in the promoter regions of overexpressed genes compared with those with low loneliness (Cole et al. 2007). In a subsequent study, Cole et al. (2011) conducted a transcript origin analysis to identify the leukocyte subset(s) that most contributed to the observed gene expression patterns in lonely individuals, finding that the transcripts were derived primarily from dendritic cells and monocytes. Given that these are both antigen-presenting cells involved in the immediate response to tissue damage, these findings suggest that chronic loneliness can shift the immune response toward a proinflammatory and a reduced antiviral response. As mentioned previously, Cole et al. (2015a) characterized rhesus macaques as high versus low in behavioral indicators of loneliness; consistent with findings in humans, rhesus macaques that were high in behavioral indicators of loneliness showed an elevated CTRA gene expression pattern and an upregulation of proinflammatory transcription factors relative to animals low in behavioral indicators of loneliness. Other studies have found that young, middle-aged, and older adults reporting greater loneliness show gene expression profiles consistent with the CTRA and proinflammatory transcription factor activity (Creswell et al. 2012; Mehl et al. 2017; Moieni et al. 2015). Importantly, in a longitudinal study with older adults, higher loneliness predicted an elevated CTRA gene expression pattern both concurrently and 1 year later (Cole et al. 2015b).

Loneliness and Antiviral Immunity

Loneliness may be particularly consequential for viral immune health. One key component of the viral response is the interferon signaling molecule, which regulates the local antiviral response and recruits macrophages and dendritic cells to the site of infection. These cells collect viral particles and present them on the cell surface to T cells and B cells to stimulate a more pronounced adaptive immune response to the viral antigen, including production of antibodies that tag the virus for destruction and proliferation of cytotoxic T cells that specifically target the viral antigen (Ivashkiv and Donlin 2014). Interferon molecules are critical to the enhancement of the viral immune response within the body. Specific evidence has begun to accumulate indicating that loneliness may shift the immune system away from viral interferon activity and toward proinflammatory activity, likely through greater activation of the SNS and subsequent increase in sympathetic fibers innervating tissue that interfaces with immune cells.

In addition to research on the CTRA gene expression pattern described earlier, studies of immune responses to viral challenge have also demonstrated reduced adaptive immune responses among lonely animals and humans. In monkeys infected with a virus analogous to HIV called the simian immunodeficiency virus (SIV), the amount of viral replication (i.e., SIV viral load) was greater among monkeys showing high versus low behavioral indicators of loneliness (Capitanio et al. 2014). The control of immune function is mediated by β-adrenergic signaling patterns, with increased innervation in lymphoid tissue in lonely and stressed animals (Sloan et al. 2008). Concomitant to this innervation is greater prevalence of SIV replication near these sympathetic nerve fibers, suggesting worse viral control as a consequence of adrenergic activity. Moreover, this is consistent with observed sympathetically driven activation of the cyclic adenosine monophosphate (cAMP)-response element binding (CREB) transcription factor among lonely individuals (Cole et al. 2007; Moieni et al. 2015).

Direct viral challenge, which can be experimentally tested using vaccines or exposure to the common cold, can also shed light on the effectiveness of the immune system to respond to a new antigen and mount an antibody response. Measuring titers generated by the immune system after vaccination to a known virus captures the efficacy of the adaptive immune system to respond to this viral challenge. In a vaccine trial that investigated viral responses to an influenza virus, higher loneliness was associated with lower titers at 1 month and 4 months after vaccination (Pressman et al. 2005). In individuals purposely exposed to a common cold virus in a controlled setting, those who reported having a reduced social network size and low social support were significantly more likely to develop symptoms of active infection after exposure (Cohen et al. 1997), suggesting a poorer viral defense. Similarly, individuals with higher loneliness reported greater cold symptoms after exposure (LeRoy et al. 2017). This work points to an important role of the social environment in modulating the immune system's response to viral challenges, with implications for both vaccine efficacy and viral defense after exposure to a virus, especially among older adults who may be more vulnerable to experiencing loneliness and have a reduced adaptive immune response due to immunosenescence. This research is particularly salient for recent SARS-CoV-2 (COVID-19) infection and vaccine efficacy (Madison et al. 2021) and suggests that, given the role of social connection in boosting immunity, interventions that target loneliness and other social factors may be particularly beneficial for individuals who are most vulnerable to poor outcomes (Cohen 2021).

Reciprocal Inflammation–Loneliness Associations

As Irwin and Cole (2011) outlined in their theoretical model, inflammatory processes can also influence behavior and perception via feedback mechanisms between the immune system and CNS. For example, an established literature in animals and humans has demonstrated that proinflammatory cytokines can induce sickness behavior, which is a coordinated behavioral response that includes symptoms such as fatigue, loss of appetite, and social withdrawal, to facilitate recovery from infection (Dantzer and Kelley 2007). Consistent with this work, emerging evidence suggests that inflammation can also influence feelings of loneliness (Moieni and Eisenberger 2018). For instance, in a longitudinal study with older adults, higher loneliness predicted an elevated CTRA gene expression profile 1 year later; however, an elevated CTRA profile also predicted higher loneliness 1 year later, suggesting a reciprocal association (Cole et al. 2015b). In addition, young adults exposed to an inflammatory challenge (i.e., endotoxin) or a placebo showed an increased proinflammatory (i.e., IL-6 and TNF-α) response to the endotoxin that was associated with increased feelings of social disconnection (Eisenberger et al. 2010). A subsequent study with the same sample found that exposure to an endotoxin was associated with increased amygdala activity to socially threatening stimuli (i.e., fear faces) along with increased feelings of social disconnection (Inagaki et al. 2012). Some evidence suggests that the inflammatory signal not only heightens amygdala reactivity to threat but also reduces dopamine reward via altered connectivity between the ventral and dorsal striatum and related ventromedial prefrontal cortex (Felger and Treadway 2017; Felger et al. 2016). These neural changes occurring via inflammatory signaling to the brain may have significant impact on social bonding and experiences of reward from social interaction (see Chapter 6, "Neurobiology of Loneliness"). Together, this work points to the reciprocal relationship between loneliness and inflammation because lonely individuals may have greater inflammatory activity that then drives further social withdrawal and threat reactivity, leading to more social isolation and feelings of loneliness.

Animal Models of Loneliness and Social Isolation

Although research with humans has identified several neuroendocrine and inflammatory pathways through which loneliness may impact health, experimental research with animal models provides an opportunity to better understand the specific neural, hormonal, and immune mechanisms involved in these pathways (Cacioppo et al. 2015). Aside from the model of loneliness that Cole et al. (2015a) developed with rhesus macaques, few studies to date have specifically investigated behavioral indicators of loneliness in animals. However, Cacioppo et al. (2015) described a large literature in which animals have been randomly assigned to normal social living conditions, socially isolated living conditions, or social living conditions separated from a preferred partner. This experimentally created a discrepancy between the animals' preferred and actual social relations that was similar to how loneliness is conceptualized in humans. For instance, one study that compared monogamous titi monkeys and polygamous squirrel monkeys found that involuntary separation from their paired mate was associated with increased plasma cortisol and behavioral signs of distress (e.g., vocalization and movement) in titi monkeys but not in squirrel monkeys (Mendoza and Mason 1986). Studies have also found that prairie voles, rodents that form enduring, selective pair bonds with a mating partner, that were isolated from their partner showed increased corticosterone levels, whereas those that were isolated from a same-sex sibling did not (Bosch et al. 2009; Grippo et al. 2007). Other studies with mice have found that repeated exposure to social threat from an aggressive conspecific was associated with increased catecholamines, glucocorticoid insensitivity, and inflammatory responses (Hanke et al. 2012; Powell et al. 2013), which may be similar to the sense of social threat observed in humans experiencing loneliness. Importantly, Cacioppo et al. (2015) noted that although the costs and benefits of sociality are common across many species, the selection of an appropriate animal model depends on the specific mechanism of interest and the nature of social relationships within a species.

Interventions for Loneliness

Another important area for future research is whether specific interventions to reduce loneliness can impact these neuroendocrine, inflammatory, and antiviral pathways. Interventions that target loneliness in older adults have been of growing interest among researchers and clinicians in the field of gerontology and geriatrics (Cattan et al. 2005; Fakoya et al. 2020; Gardiner et al. 2018; O'Rourke et al. 2018), and interventions have also been developed for young adults and individuals with mental and physical health conditions (Eccles and Qualter 2021). Masi et al. (2011) conducted a meta-analysis investigating the efficacy of interventions specifically targeting loneliness in children, adolescents, and adults. The authors identified four types of interventions that aimed to increase opportunities for social contact, enhance social support, improve social skills, and address maladaptive social cognition. Findings from this meta-analysis suggested that the interventions had a small but significant effect on loneliness and that the largest improvement in loneliness was observed for interventions that addressed maladaptive cognition (e.g., within a cognitive-behavioral therapy framework) (Masi et al. 2011). Another review suggested that interventions that focused on changing cognitions were the most promising for individuals with mental health problems (Mann et al. 2017).

Although systematic reviews of this literature suggest that most interventions have some effect on reducing loneliness, the quality of the evidence is not strong, and research is needed to better understand moderators of treatment effectiveness (e.g., which treatments work best for whom and in which context) (Fakoya et al. 2020; Gardiner et al. 2018; Mann et al. 2017; Masi et al. 2011). (Please see Chapter 8, "Interventions for Loneliness in Younger People"; Chapter 9, "Interventions for Loneliness in Older Adults"; and Chapter 10, "Community-Based Interventions for Loneliness.")

A few studies to date have investigated the effectiveness of behavioral interventions for reducing both loneliness and inflammatory biology. In a recent intervention study with a small sample, older adults who had a chronic illness and reported chronic loneliness participated in either a group-based loneliness intervention (Loneliness Intervention using Story Theory to Enhance Nursing sensitive outcomes, or LISTEN) that used narrative and cognitive restructuring techniques or a healthy aging education control group. Those who completed the intervention showed a trend toward decreases in loneliness compared to those in the control group, although corresponding decreases in expression of proinflammatory genes (i.e., *IL2, IL6*) did not reach the threshold for statistical significance (Theeke et al. 2016). Although it did not directly target loneliness, a pilot study by Creswell et al. (2012) showed that older adults who participated in a mindfulness-based stress reduction program that included mindfulness meditation, yoga, and exercises to increase awareness of momentary experiences reported larger decreases in loneliness and showed decreasing proinflammatory gene expression compared with a waitlist control group (Creswell et al. 2012).

Another pilot study tested the effects of a 9-month Generation Xchange program, an intergenerational helping intervention that trains and places older adult volunteers in elementary school classrooms to aid students' academic development and address behavioral issues (Seeman et al. 2020). Although the intervention did not specifically enroll older adults high in loneliness, it found that the intervention increased levels of eudaimonic well-being and decreased CTRA gene expression patterns. Importantly, eudaimonic well-being—which has been defined as having a sense of meaning or purpose in life—has been inversely associated with loneliness and accounted for much of the effects of loneliness on CTRA in other research (Cole et al. 2015b), suggesting that it may be a promising target for future interventions aimed at reducing loneliness and its biological sequelae.

Case Vignette

Tom is a 72-year-old male who presented in a primary care setting with a 10-year history of poorly controlled type 2 diabetes and cardiovascular disease. His symptoms had worsened in recent years to include pain and tingling (neuropathy) in his hands and feet, blurry vision, and lightheadedness that he reported had contributed to a recent motor vehicle accident and led him to seek medical care. Tom was employed part-time as a handyman and lived alone. He had an estranged relationship with his adult son, who lived several hours away, and otherwise had occasional interactions with a few co-workers and neighbors in his apartment complex. Tom also explained that over the past year his symptoms had made it difficult for him to work, and he was spending more time inside his apartment. When asked about other symptoms he might be experiencing, he endorsed feeling less interested in his hobbies, such as gardening or walking, and in socializing, explaining that "everything feels like a chore." Tom explained that he relied mostly on processed and convenience foods for his meals and often spent hours in his recliner watching television and getting up only to prepare a frozen dinner. He expressed ambivalence about making dietary changes and increasing physical activity, explaining that he was just too tired.

Tom was open to speaking with a clinical psychologist about the anhedonia and fatigue he was experiencing and was referred for psychotherapy. During the initial psychotherapy session, Tom expressed that he was bothered by how much his symptoms had limited his daily functioning and how isolated he felt at home alone. He explained that he wanted to have more meaningful relationships with people, including his son, but he did not know how and did not want to be a burden to others. The early focus of psychotherapy was to identify and better understand how Tom's feelings of loneliness, depressive symptoms, and worsening of his diabetes and cardiovascular disease were interrelated and how inflammation may play a role in each. The psychologist worked with Tom to develop a treatment plan that included cognitive-behavioral therapy to address his thoughts and behaviors related to his health, his social interactions, and his relationship with his son and motivational interviewing to explore making dietary and lifestyle changes to improve his health.

After several sessions of psychotherapy, Tom had an important insight that he wanted to contribute something positive and leave behind a legacy in the remaining years of his life. The psychologist spoke with Tom about the concepts of generativity and eudaimonic well-being, which have both been associated with decreased loneliness and improved mental and physical health. This became his motivation for restarting his garden, so that he could share his vegetables with neighbors and eat healthier himself, and for reaching out to his son in an effort to repair their relationship. As Tom made progress in these goals, his depression symptoms also began to improve, and he became more actively engaged socially and in the management of his diabetes and cardiovascular disease.

Future Directions

Sympathetic Innervation of the Bone Marrow

A growing body of research with animals suggests that SNS activation may influence the composition of the leukocyte population in circulation through

SNS innervation of the bone marrow microenvironment. For instance, one impressive study found that mice exposed to chronic variable stressors had increased levels of noradrenaline, augmented colony-forming capacity indicative of increased progenitor cell proliferation, and higher numbers of hematopoietic stem cells in the bone marrow compared with those not exposed (Heidt et al. 2014). In addition, stressed mice showed an increased proportion of total leukocytes, neutrophils, and immature monocytes in their blood and bone marrow compared with non-stressed mice. Consistent with these findings, another study found that, relative to mice in the control group, mice exposed to repeated social threat from an aggressive conspecific showed increased expression of a growth factor involved in blood stem cell proliferation that led to an increased production of myeloid lineage white blood cells and consequent elevations in immature monocytes and granulocytes in the blood, spleen, and bone marrow (Powell et al. 2013). These effects were mediated by SNS activity and could be blocked by pharmacological blockade of β-adrenergic receptors. As a result of SNS-mediated increases in circulating myeloid progenitor cells, the spleen is colonized to form a temporary white blood cell production environment to supplement the bone marrow (McKim et al. 2018). As mentioned previously, Cole and colleagues (Chun et al. 2017; Cole et al. 2015a; Sloan et al. 2006, 2007) conducted several studies using a social threat model in rhesus macaques, whom they randomized to socialize for 5 weeks with either a continuously changing group of novel social partners (chronic social threat) or a stable group of social partners. They found that those who were exposed to chronic social threat showed increased prevalence of immature monocytes in circulation (Cole et al. 2015a) and enhanced density of SNS nerve fibers in axillary lymph nodes (Sloan et al. 2007), which was associated with reduced transcription of antiviral genes (Chun et al. 2017; Sloan et al. 2006) and a related reduction in resistance to a chronic viral infection (Cole et al. 2015a). Although studies that examine the impact of loneliness on SNS innervation of the bone marrow are more challenging to conduct in humans, this is an important question for future research employing both animal and human models, with important implications for disease.

Novel Biological Aging Pathways

Another rapidly developing area of research investigates the impact of chronic stress and the exposure to the repeated activation of the stress response system on biological aging pathways, including accumulation of DNA damage, telomere length shortening, mitochondrial dysfunction, and increased cellular senescence (Entringer and Epel 2020; Kirkland and Tchkonia 2017; Rentscher et al. 2020b; Robles and Carroll 2011). These hallmarks of biological aging are thought to be drivers of age-related diseases such as diabetes, arthritis, cancer, dementia, and cardiovascular disease (López-Otín et al. 2013) and to have significant implications within the immune system. Chronic stress, through prolonged or repeated activation of the SNS and release of catecholamines, can increase the production of oxidants and DNA damage within cells (Aschbacher et al. 2013; Flint et al. 2005, 2007; Hara et al. 2011; Knickelbein et al. 2008). If unresolved, excess DNA damage can result in cellular senescence and accelerate the shortening of telomeres (the protective caps at the end of chromosomes that protect the DNA), which can also lead to senescence if telomeres reach a critically short length (Blackburn 2000; Campisi 2005; Choi et al. 2008; Fumagalli et al. 2012). Cellular senescence is a state of permanent cell growth arrest associated with heightened release of proinflammatory factors, including cytokines, chemokines, and growth factors, termed the *senescence-associated secretory phenotype* (SASP). Importantly, the SASP is thought to be a source of the increased inflammation observed with older age (i.e., "inflammaging") and to contribute to age-related disease (Campisi and D'Adda Di Fagagna 2007; Collado et al. 2007; Coppé et al. 2010; Effros et al. 2005; Rodier and Campisi 2011). Immunosenescence has increasingly been identified as a factor impacting susceptibility to severe infection from viral exposures, which is particularly relevant for SARS-CoV-2 (COVID-19) and vaccination immunity (Akbar and Gilroy 2020). Accelerated immune senescence via these biological aging pathways could be a consequence of social isolation, further altering risk among vulnerable groups. The SASP may also be a source of chronic inflammation that drives sickness behavior, including social withdrawal and amplification of feelings of loneliness, although this remains to be empirically tested.

Only three studies to date have examined associations between loneliness and telomere length as a marker of biological aging, with mixed findings, although several studies have reported links between social relationships and telomere length (Rentscher et al. 2020b). For instance, one study found that former prisoners of war who reported greater loneliness after deployment had shorter leukocyte telomere length 24 years later (Stein et al. 2018); however, two other studies with older males and older adults with depression did not find an association (Rius-Ottenheim et al. 2012; Schaakxs et al. 2016). Another study with middle-aged parents found that higher relationship closeness with one's spouse buffered the effects of perceived stress on gene expression of p16^{INK4a} (e.g., *CDKN2A*), a robust marker of cellular senescence (Rentscher et al. 2020a). Based on these initial studies and growing evidence from animal and human research that other forms of chronic stress can impact several biological aging pathways (Entringer and Epel 2020), research that examines whether and how loneliness influences these pathways may provide important insights into aging, health, and disease and novel targets for intervention.

Language-Based Measures of Loneliness

Recent developments in natural language processing methods have also introduced innovative metrics to assess loneliness in humans. For instance, one study interviewed older adults about their experience of loneliness (e.g., "Do you ever feel lonely? What does loneliness feel like for you?") and used artificial intelligence and machine learning approaches to identify subtle variations in the participants' sentiment (e.g., level of agreement with the current conversation) and expressed emotions (e.g., sadness, fear) during the interview that corresponded with but were distinct from self-reported loneliness (Badal et al. 2021). Individuals who acknowledged feeling lonely were more likely to express sadness in their responses to the questions, and machine learning could accurately predict whether participants endorsed feeling lonely based solely on features of their natural speech during the interview. Another study used a naturalistic observation tool called the Electronically Activated Recorder to investigate participants' natural speech during daily social interactions, finding that their total language output and patterns of function-word use covaried with CTRA gene expression patterns (Mehl et al. 2017). Although it was not the primary focus of the study, the authors also found that individuals reporting higher loneliness used fewer prepositions (e.g., to, with, above), spent less time speaking to others, and spent more time alone. The integration of these innovative language-based metrics of loneliness, which are thought to provide behavioral indicators of more implicit psychological processes, with biological assessments of neuroendocrine and inflammatory pathways represents an exciting direction for future research.

Summary

One general pathway through which loneliness may be associated with increased health risk involves CNS-mediated alterations in neural and endocrine activity that subsequently affect immune function in ways that may both promote the development and progression of chronic disease and reciprocally feed back to the brain to amplify and prolong experiences of social threat and loneliness (Figure 7–1). Among the peripheral neuroendocrine mechanisms involved, current evidence for SNS activity is limited, with human and animal studies suggesting that loneliness is associated with increased urinary levels of norepinephrine, a catecholamine produced by the SNS during the stress response. There is also some evidence from animal

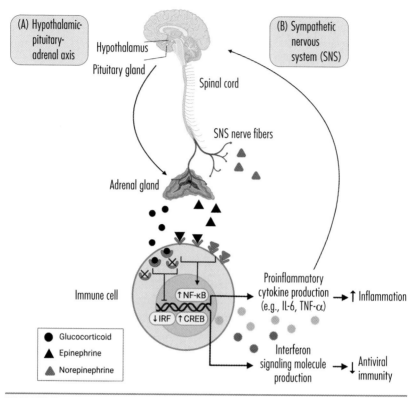

FIGURE 7–1. **Neuroendocrine and inflammatory mechanisms in loneliness.**

When the body perceives an environmental threat such as loneliness, the HPA axis (A) releases glucocorticoids (e.g., cortisol) into peripheral circulation that interact with GRs in immune cells to regulate expression of immune response genes. GR activation can have an anti-inflammatory effect by suppressing NF-κB-mediated transcription of proinflammatory genes; however, prolonged activation is thought to result in reduced sensitivity of GRs to cortisol's anti-inflammatory effects, adding to increased inflammation. GR activation can also suppress IRF-mediated transcription of type I interferon genes, leading to decreased antiviral immunity. Similarly, in response to threat the SNS (B) releases norepinephrine from nerve fibers into organs and tissues and stimulates the adrenal glands to release epinephrine into circulation that interacts with adrenergic receptors on the surface of immune cells to activate proinflammatory transcription factors CREB and NF-κB and increase transcription of proinflammatory genes, leading to increased inflammation. Adrenergic receptor activation can also suppress IRF-mediated transcription of type I interferon genes, leading to decreased antiviral immunity. Proinflammatory cytokines may also reciprocally feed back to the brain to amplify and prolong experiences of social threat and loneliness.

CREB=cyclic adenosine monophosphate–response element binding protein; GR= glucocorticoid receptor; HPA=hypothalamic-pituitary-adrenal; IL=interleukin; IRF= interferon response factor; NF-κB=nuclear factor-κB; TNF=tumor necrosis factor.
Source.   Figure created with BioRender.com.

models that behavioral indicators of loneliness can influence the composition of the leukocyte population in circulation by increasing the proportion of immature classical monocytes. The link between loneliness and HPA axis activity has the most well-developed literature of all the pathways reviewed. Although researchers have used several approaches to measure glucocorticoid levels, the strongest evidence comes from studies of the CAR in which loneliness is associated with a higher CAR in young and middle-aged adults but a lower CAR in older adults, which may have detrimental effects on health, including greater wear and tear and poorer inflammatory regulation by cortisol. Surprisingly few studies link loneliness to peripheral protein markers of inflammation such as CRP or IL-6, with investigations of CRP yielding inconsistent findings and a handful of experimental studies demonstrating that individuals high in loneliness show an elevated inflammatory response to acute psychological and physiological (e.g., endotoxin, vaccine) stress.

A growing body of research has also investigated transcriptome dynamics in humans and animals, finding that loneliness is associated with increased proinflammatory and decreased glucocorticoid receptors and antiviral gene expression and transcription control pathways (Eisenberger and Cole 2012; Leschak and Eisenberger 2019). Research on the CTRA has the advantage of being driven by massively multivariate measures of immune regulation at the genomic level, which may help to disentangle the effects of loneliness on inflammatory processes. Accumulating evidence from a few human and animal studies also suggests that loneliness is associated with changes in white blood cell production and circulation that may increase vulnerability to inflammation-related chronic disease while simultaneously reducing immune response to viral challenge and vaccinations. Several gaps in this area remain, including a better understanding of the CNS mechanisms that connect the experience of loneliness to changes in peripheral neural and endocrine function, and the distinct biological correlates of loneliness in blood versus solid tissue environments (which do not necessarily correlate with one another and may show distinct associations with loneliness).

Implications for the biology of health and disease production also remain to be explored more fully, although a growing literature has connected experiences of loneliness and social isolation with reduced antiviral immunity (Cohen 2021; LeRoy et al. 2017; Madison et al. 2021; Pressman et al. 2005) and accelerated cancer progression and metastasis (Bower et al. 2018; Lutgendorf et al. 2011, 2012, 2018, 2020). Understanding how loneliness alters immune response and identifying behavioral and pharmacological strategies to ameliorate the negative sequelae have important consequences for population health in this era of renewed focus on host resistance to viral infection and vaccination responses. Finally, growing evidence also suggests that inflammation can reciprocally influence perceptions of threat and social withdrawal driving further loneliness, making intervening to stop the feedforward loop critical for public health. Further evidence is needed to better characterize these CNS-immune feedback mechanisms and develop new strategies for breaking the reciprocal relationship between loneliness and inflammation.

KEY POINTS

- Loneliness is associated with the activation of several neuroendocrine and inflammatory pathways thought to be evolutionarily adaptive for short-term survival but detrimental for long-term health, increasing risk for morbidity and early mortality.

- Loneliness may influence leukocyte composition through sympathetic nervous system innervation of the bone marrow, thereby increasing the proportion of immature monocytes in circulation and contributing to systemic inflammation.

- Loneliness is associated with a higher cortisol awakening response (CAR) in young and middle-aged adults but a lower CAR in older adults, which may have detrimental effects on health, including greater wear and tear and poorer inflammatory regulation by cortisol.

- Loneliness is associated with a shift in the transcriptome toward increased proinflammatory and decreased glucocorticoid receptor and antiviral gene expression and transcription control pathways.

- There is also evidence that inflammation can reciprocally influence CNS perceptions of threat and social withdrawal, driving further loneliness, making intervening to stop the feedforward loop critical for public health.

Suggested Readings

Cacioppo JT, Cacioppo S: Loneliness in the modern age: an evolutionary theory of loneliness (ETL). Adv Exp Soc Psychol 58:127–197, 2018

Cole SW, Capitanio JP, Chun K, et al: Myeloid differentiation architecture of leukocyte transcriptome dynamics in perceived social isolation. Proc Natl Acad Sci USA 112(49):15142–15147, 2015

Irwin MR, Cole SW: Reciprocal regulation of the neural and innate immune systems. Nat Rev Immunol 11(9):625–632, 2011

Moieni M, Eisenberger NI: Effects of inflammation on social processes and implications for health. Ann NY Acad Sci 1428(1):5–13, 2018 29806109

Steptoe A, Owen N, Kunz-Ebrecht SR, Brydon L: Loneliness and neuro-endocrine, cardiovascular, and inflammatory stress responses in middle-aged men and women. Psychoneuroendocrinology 29:593–611, 2004

References

Adam EK, Hawkley LC, Kudielka BM, Cacioppo JT: Day-to-day dynamics of ex-perience-cortisol associations in a population-based sample of older adults. Proc Natl Acad Sci USA 103(45):17058–17063, 2006 17075058

Akbar AN, Gilroy DW: Aging immunity may exacerbate COVID-19. Science 369(6501):256–257, 2020 32675364

Aschbacher K, O'Donovan A, Wolkowitz OM, et al: Good stress, bad stress and ox-idative stress: insights from anticipatory cortisol reactivity. Psychoneuroendo-crinology 38(9):1698–1708, 2013 23490070

Badal VD, Graham SA, Depp CA, et al: Prediction of loneliness in older adults us-ing natural language processing: exploring sex differences in speech. Am J Geri-atr Psychiatry 29(8):853–866, 2021 33039266

Balter LJT, Raymond JE, Aldred S, et al: Loneliness in healthy young adults pre-dicts inflammatory responsiveness to a mild immune challenge in vivo. Brain Be-hav Immun 82:298–301, 2019 31476413

Blackburn EH: Telomere states and cell fates. Nature 408(6808):53–56, 2000 11081503

Bosch OJ, Nair HP, Ahern TH, et al: The CRF system mediates increased passive stress-coping behavior following the loss of a bonded partner in a monogamous rodent. Neuropsychopharmacology 34(6):1406–1415, 2009 18923404

Bower JE, Shiao SL, Sullivan P, et al: Prometastatic molecular profiles in breast tumors from socially isolated women. JNCI Cancer Spectr 2(3):pky029, 2018 30057973

Buchman AS, Boyle PA, Wilson RS, et al: Loneliness and the rate of motor decline in old age: the Rush Memory and Aging Project, a community-based cohort study. BMC Geriatr 10(1):77, 2010 20969786

Cacioppo JT, Cacioppo S: Loneliness in the modern age: an evolutionary theory of loneliness (ETL). Adv Exp Soc Psychol 58:127–197, 2018

Cacioppo JT, Hawkley LC: Perceived social isolation and cognition. Trends Cogn Sci 13(10):447–454, 2009 19726219

Cacioppo JT, Ernst JM, Burleson MH, et al: Lonely traits and concomitant physi-ological processes: the MacArthur social neuroscience studies. Int J Psycho-physiol 35(2–3):143–154, 2000 10677643

Cacioppo JT, Hughes ME, Waite LJ, et al: Loneliness as a specific risk factor for depressive symptoms: cross-sectional and longitudinal analyses. Psychol Aging 21(1):140–151, 2006 16594799

Cacioppo JT, Hawkley LC, Thisted RA: Perceived social isolation makes me sad: 5-year cross-lagged analyses of loneliness and depressive symptomatology in the Chicago Health, Aging, and Social Relations Study. Psychol Aging 25(2):453–463, 2010 20545429

Cacioppo JT, Cacioppo S, Cole SW, et al: Loneliness across phylogeny and a call for comparative studies and animal models. Perspect Psychol Sci 10(2):202–212, 2015 25910390

Campisi J: Senescent cells, tumor suppression, and organismal aging: good citizens, bad neighbors. Cell 120(4):513–522, 2005 15734683

Campisi J, D'Adda Di Fagagna F: Cellular senescence: when bad things happen to good cells. Nat Rev Mol Cell Biol 8(9):729–740, 2007 17667954

Capitanio JP, Hawkley LC, Cole SW, Cacioppo JT: A behavioral taxonomy of loneliness in humans and rhesus monkeys (Macaca mulatta). PLoS One 9(10):e110307, 2014 25354040

Cattan M, White M, Bond J, Learmouth A: Preventing social isolation and loneliness among older people: a systematic review of health promotion interventions. Ageing Soc 25(1):41–67, 2005

Choi J, Fauce SR, Effros RB: Reduced telomerase activity in human T lymphocytes exposed to cortisol. Brain Behav Immun 22(4):600–605, 2008 18222063

Chun K, Capitanio JP, Lamkin DM, et al: Social regulation of the lymph node transcriptome in rhesus macaques (Macaca mulatta). Psychoneuroendocrinology 76:107–113, 2017 27902946

Cohen S: Psychosocial vulnerabilities to upper respiratory infectious illness: implications for susceptibility to coronavirus disease 2019 (COVID-19). Perspect Psychol Sci 16(1):161–174, 2021 32640177

Cohen S, Doyle WJ, Skoner DP, et al: Social ties and susceptibility to the common cold. JAMA 277(24):1940–1944, 1997 9200634

Cole SW: Social regulation of leukocyte homeostasis: the role of glucocorticoid sensitivity. Brain Behav Immun 22(7):1049–1055, 2008 18394861

Cole SW: Human social genomics. PLoS Genet 10(8):e1004601, 2014 25166010

Cole SW: The conserved transcriptional response to adversity. Curr Opin Behav Sci 28:31–37, 2019 31592179

Cole SW, Yan W, Galic Z, et al: Expression-based monitoring of transcription factor activity: the TELiS database. Bioinformatics 21(6):803–810, 2005 15374858

Cole SW, Hawkley LC, Arevalo JM, et al: Social regulation of gene expression in human leukocytes. Genome Biol 8(9):R189, 2007 17854483

Cole SW, Hawkley LC, Arevalo JM, et al: Transcript origin analysis identifies antigen-presenting cells as primary targets of socially regulated gene expression in leukocytes. Proc Natl Acad Sci USA 108(7):3080–3085, 2011 21300872

Cole SW, Capitanio JP, Chun K, et al: Myeloid differentiation architecture of leukocyte transcriptome dynamics in perceived social isolation. Proc Natl Acad Sci USA 112(49):15142–15147, 2015a 26598672

Cole SW, Levine ME, Arevalo JM, et al: Loneliness, eudaimonia, and the human conserved transcriptional response to adversity. Psychoneuroendocrinology 62:11–17, 2015b 26246388

Collado M, Blasco MA, Serrano M: Cellular senescence in cancer and aging. Cell 130(2):223–233, 2007 17662938

Coppé J-P, Desprez P-Y, Krtolica A, Campisi J: The senescence-associated secretory phenotype: the dark side of tumor suppression. Annu Rev Pathol 5(1):99–118, 2010 20078217

Creswell JD, Irwin MR, Burklund LJ, et al: Mindfulness-based stress reduction training reduces loneliness and pro-inflammatory gene expression in older adults: a small randomized controlled trial. Brain Behav Immun 26(7):1095–1101, 2012 22820409

Dantzer R, Kelley KW: Twenty years of research on cytokine-induced sickness behavior. Brain Behav Immun 21(2):153–160, 2007 17088043

Dantzer R, O'Connor JC, Freund GG, et al: From inflammation to sickness and depression: when the immune system subjugates the brain. Nat Rev Neurosci 9(1):46–56, 2008 18073775

Doane LD, Adam EK: Loneliness and cortisol: momentary, day-to-day, and trait associations. Psychoneuroendocrinology 35(3):430–441, 2010 19744794

Drake EC, Sladek MR, Doane LD: Daily cortisol activity, loneliness, and coping efficacy in late adolescence: a longitudinal study of the transition to college. Int J Behav Dev 40(4):334–345, 2016 28979055

Eccles AM, Qualter P: Review: Alleviating loneliness in young people: a meta-analysis of interventions. Child Adolesc Ment Health 26(1):17–33, 2021 32406165

Effros RB, Dagarag M, Spaulding C, Man J: The role of CD8+ T-cell replicative senescence in human aging. Immunol Rev 205(27):147–157, 2005 15882351

Eisenberger NI, Cole SW: Social neuroscience and health: neurophysiological mechanisms linking social ties with physical health. Nat Neurosci 15(5):669–674, 2012 22504347

Eisenberger NI, Inagaki TK, Mashal NM, Irwin MR: Inflammation and social experience: an inflammatory challenge induces feelings of social disconnection in addition to depressed mood. Brain Behav Immun 24(4):558–563, 2010 20043983

Elenkov IJ, Wilder RL, Chrousos GP, Vizi ES: The sympathetic nerve: an integrative interface between two supersystems: the brain and the immune system. Pharmacol Rev 52(4):595–638, 2000

Entringer S, Epel ES: The stress field ages: a close look into cellular aging processes. Psychoneuroendocrinology 113:104537, 2020 32085926

Fakoya OA, McCorry NK, Donnelly M: Loneliness and social isolation interventions for older adults: a scoping review of reviews. BMC Public Health 20(1):129, 2020 32054474

Felger JC, Treadway MT: Inflammation effects on motivation and motor activity: role of dopamine. Neuropsychopharmacology 42(1):216–241, 2017 27480574

Felger JC, Li Z, Haroon E, et al: Inflammation is associated with decreased functional connectivity within corticostriatal reward circuitry in depression. Mol Psychiatry 21(10):1358–1365, 2016 26552591

Flint MS, Carroll JE, Jenkins FJ, et al: Genomic profiling of restraint stress-induced alterations in mouse T lymphocytes. J Neuroimmunol 167(1–2):34–44, 2005 16026860

Flint MS, Baum A, Chambers WH, Jenkins FJ: Induction of DNA damage, alteration of DNA repair and transcriptional activation by stress hormones. Psychoneuroendocrinology 32(5):470–479, 2007 17459596

Fumagalli M, Rossiello F, Clerici M, et al: Telomeric DNA damage is irreparable and causes persistent DNA-damage-response activation. Nat Cell Biol 14(4):355–365, 2012 22426077

Gardiner C, Geldenhuys G, Gott M: Interventions to reduce social isolation and loneliness among older people: an integrative review. Health Soc Care Community 26(2):147–157, 2018 27413007

Grippo AJ, Gerena D, Huang J, et al: Social isolation induces behavioral and neuroendocrine disturbances relevant to depression in female and male prairie voles. Psychoneuroendocrinology 32(8–10):966–980, 2007 17825994

Hackett RA, Hamer M, Endrighi R, et al: Loneliness and stress-related inflammatory and neuroendocrine responses in older men and women. Psychoneuroendocrinology 37(11):1801–1809, 2012 22503139

Hanke ML, Powell ND, Stiner LM, et al: Beta adrenergic blockade decreases the immunomodulatory effects of social disruption stress. Brain Behav Immun 26(7):1150–1159, 2012 22841997

Hara MR, Kovacs JJ, Whalen EJ, et al: A stress response pathway regulates DNA damage through beta2-adrenoreceptors and beta-arrestin-1. Nature 477(7364):349–353, 2011 21857681

Hart BL: Biological basis of the behavior of sick animals. Neurosci Biobehav Rev 12(2):123–137, 1988 3050629

Hawkley LC, Masi CM, Berry JD, Cacioppo JT: Loneliness is a unique predictor of age-related differences in systolic blood pressure. Psychol Aging 21(1):152–164, 2006 16594800

Heidt T, Sager HB, Courties G, et al: Chronic variable stress activates hematopoietic stem cells. Nat Med 20(7):754–758, 2014

Holt-Lunstad J, Smith TB: Loneliness and social isolation as risk factors for CVD: implications for evidence-based patient care and scientific inquiry. Heart 102(13):987–989, 2016 27091845

Holt-Lunstad J, Smith TB, Baker M, et al: Loneliness and social isolation as risk factors for mortality: a meta-analytic review. Perspect Psychol Sci 10(2):227–237, 2015

Holt-Lunstad J, Robles TF, Sbarra DA: Advancing social connection as a public health priority in the United States. Am Psychol 72(6):517–530, 2017 28880099

Inagaki TK, Muscatell KA, Irwin MR, et al: Inflammation selectively enhances amygdala activity to socially threatening images. Neuroimage 59(4):3222–3226, 2012 22079507

Irwin MR, Cole SW: Reciprocal regulation of the neural and innate immune systems. Nat Rev Immunol 11(9):625–632, 2011 21818124

Ivashkiv LB, Donlin LT: Regulation of type I interferon responses. Nat Rev Immunol 14(1):36–49, 2014 24362405

Jaremka LM, Fagundes CP, Peng J, et al: Loneliness promotes inflammation during acute stress. Psychol Sci 24(7):1089–1097, 2013 23630220

Johar H, Atasoy S, Bidlingmaier M, et al: Married but lonely: impact of poor marital quality on diurnal cortisol patterns in older people: findings from the cross-sectional KORA-Age study. Stress 24(1):36–43, 2021 32166997

Kiecolt-Glaser JK, Ricker D, George J, et al: Urinary cortisol levels, cellular immunocompetency, and loneliness in psychiatric inpatients. Psychosom Med 46(1):15–23, 1984 6701251

Kirkland JL, Tchkonia T: Cellular senescence: a translational perspective. EBioMedicine 21:21–28, 2017 28416161

Knickelbein KZ, Flint M, Jenkins F, Baum A: Psychological stress and oxidative damage in lymphocytes of aerobically fit and unfit individuals. J Appl Biobehav Res 13(1):1–19, 2008

Lai JCL, Leung MOY, Lee DYH, et al: Loneliness and diurnal salivary cortisol in emerging adults. Int J Mol Sci 19(7):1944, 2018 29970811

LeRoy AS, Murdock KW, Jaremka LM, et al: Loneliness predicts self-reported cold symptoms after a viral challenge. Health Psychol 36(5):512–520, 2017 28358524

Leschak CJ, Eisenberger NI: Two distinct immune pathways linking social relationships with health: inflammatory and antiviral processes. Psychosom Med 81(8):711–719, 2019 31600173

López-Otín C, Blasco MA, Partridge L, et al: The hallmarks of aging. Cell 153(6):1194–1217, 2013 23746838

Lutgendorf SK, Andersen BL: Biobehavioral approaches to cancer progression and survival: mechanisms and interventions. Am Psychol 70(2):186–197, 2015 25730724

Lutgendorf SK, DeGeest K, Dahmoush L, et al: Social isolation is associated with elevated tumor norepinephrine in ovarian carcinoma patients. Brain Behav Immun 25(2):250–255, 2011 20955777

Lutgendorf SK, De Geest K, Bender D, et al: Social influences on clinical outcomes of patients with ovarian cancer. J Clin Oncol 30(23):2885–2890, 2012 22802321

Lutgendorf SK, Thaker PH, Arevalo JM, et al: Biobehavioral modulation of the exosome transcriptome in ovarian carcinoma. Cancer 124(3):580–586, 2018 29112229

Lutgendorf SK, Penedo F, Goodheart MJ, et al: Epithelial-mesenchymal transition polarization in ovarian carcinomas from patients with high social isolation. Cancer 126(19):4407–4413, 2020 32691853

Madison AA, Shrout MR, Renna ME, Kiecolt-Glaser JK: Psychological and behavioral predictors of vaccine efficacy: considerations for COVID-19. Perspect Psychol Sci 16(2):191–203, 2021 33501900

Mann F, Bone JK, Lloyd-Evans B, et al: A life less lonely: the state of the art in interventions to reduce loneliness in people with mental health problems. Soc Psychiatry Psychiatr Epidemiol 52(6):627–638, 2017 28528389

Masi CM, Chen HY, Hawkley LC, Cacioppo JT: A meta-analysis of interventions to reduce loneliness. Pers Soc Psychol Rev 15(3):219–266, 2011 20716644

McKim DB, Yin W, Wang Y, et al: Social stress mobilizes hematopoietic stem cells to establish persistent splenic myelopoiesis. Cell Rep 25(9):2552–2562, 2018 30485819

Mehl MR, Raison CL, Pace TWW, et al: Natural language indicators of differential gene regulation in the human immune system. Proc Natl Acad Sci USA 114(47):12554–12559, 2017 29109260

Mendoza SP, Mason WA: Contrasting responses to intruders and to involuntary separation by monogamous and polygynous New World monkeys. Physiol Behav 38(6):795–801, 1986 3823197

Mezuk B, Choi M, DeSantis AS, et al: Loneliness, depression, and inflammation: evidence from the multi-ethnic study of atherosclerosis. PLoS One 11(7):e0158056, 2016 27367428

Miller AH, Maletic V, Raison CL: Inflammation and its discontents: the role of cytokines in the pathophysiology of major depression. Biol Psychiatry 65(9):732–741, 2009 19150053

Moieni M, Eisenberger NI: Effects of inflammation on social processes and implications for health. Ann N Y Acad Sci 1428(1):5–13, 2018 29806109

Moieni M, Irwin MR, Jevtic I, et al: Trait sensitivity to social disconnection enhances pro-inflammatory responses to a randomized controlled trial of endotoxin. Psychoneuroendocrinology 62:336–342, 2015 26360770

Nersesian PV, Han HR, Yenokyan G, et al: Loneliness in middle age and biomarkers of systemic inflammation: findings from midlife in the United States. Soc Sci Med 209:174–181, 2018 29735350

O'Connor DB, Thayer JF, Vedhara K: Stress and health: a review of psychobiological processes. Annu Rev Psychol 72:663–688, 2021 32886587

Okamura H, Tsuda A, Matsuishi T: The relationship between perceived loneliness and cortisol awakening responses on work days and weekends. Jpn Psychol Res 53(2):113–120, 2011

O'Luanaigh C, O'Connell H, Chin AV, et al: Loneliness and vascular biomarkers: the Dublin Healthy Ageing Study. Int J Geriatr Psychiatry 27(1):83–88, 2012 21370279

O'Rourke HM, Collins L, Sidani S: Interventions to address social connectedness and loneliness for older adults: a scoping review. BMC Geriatrics 18(1):214, 2018 30219034

Pavela G, Kim YI, Salvy S-J: Additive effects of obesity and loneliness on C-reactive protein. PLoS One 13(11):e0206092, 2018 30439985

Powell ND, Sloan EK, Bailey MT, et al: Social stress up-regulates inflammatory gene expression in the leukocyte transcriptome via beta-adrenergic induction of myelopoiesis. Proc Natl Acad Sci USA 110(41):16574–16579, 2013 24062448

Pressman SD, Cohen S, Miller GE, et al: Loneliness, social network size, and immune response to influenza vaccination in college freshmen. Health Psychol 24(3):297–306, 2005 15898866

Rentscher KE, Carroll JE, Cole SW, et al: Relationship closeness buffers the effects of perceived stress on transcriptomic indicators of cellular stress and biological aging marker p16INK4a. Aging (Albany NY) 12(16):16476–16490, 2020a 32712602

Rentscher KE, Carroll JE, Mitchell C: Psychosocial stressors and telomere length: a current review of the science. Annu Rev Public Health 41:223–245, 2020b 31900099

Rius-Ottenheim N, Houben JMJ, Kromhout D, et al: Telomere length and mental well-being in elderly men from the Netherlands and Greece. Behav Genet 42(2):278–286, 2012 21870178

Robles TF, Carroll JE: Restorative biological processes and health. Soc Personal Psychol Compass 5(8):518–537, 2011 21927619

Rodier F, Campisi J: Four faces of cellular senescence. J Cell Biol 192(4):547–556, 2011 21321098

Rueggeberg R, Wrosch C, Miller GE, McDade TW: Associations between health-related self-protection, diurnal cortisol, and C-reactive protein in lonely older adults. Psychosom Med 74(9):937–944, 2012 23115346

Schaakxs R, Wielaard I, Verhoeven JE, et al: Early and recent psychosocial stress and telomere length in older adults. Int Psychogeriatr 28(3):405–413, 2016 26265356

Schutter N, Holwerda TJ, Stek ML, et al: Loneliness in older adults is associated with diminished cortisol output. J Psychosom Res 95:19–25, 2017 28314545

Seeman T, Merkin SS, Goldwater D, Cole SW: Intergenerational mentoring, eudaimonic well-being and gene regulation in older adults: a pilot study. Psychoneuroendocrinology 111:104468, 2020 31589939

Segerstrom SC, Miller GE: Psychological stress and the human immune system: a meta-analytic study of 30 years of inquiry. Psychol Bull 130(4):601–630, 2004 15250815

Shankar A, McMunn A, Banks J, Steptoe A: Loneliness, social isolation, and behavioral and biological health indicators in older adults. Health Psychol 30(4):377–385, 2011 21534675

Sladek MR, Doane LD: Daily diary reports of social connection, objective sleep, and the cortisol awakening response during adolescents' first year of college. J Youth Adolesc 44(2):298–316, 2015 25537099

Sloan EK, Tarara RP, Capitanio JP, Cole SW: Enhanced replication of simian immunodeficiency virus adjacent to catecholaminergic varicosities in primate lymph nodes. J Virol 80(9):4326–4335, 2006 16611891

Sloan EK, Capitanio JP, Tarara RP, et al: Social stress enhances sympathetic innervation of primate lymph nodes: mechanisms and implications for viral pathogenesis. J Neurosci 27(33):8857–8865, 2007 17699667

Sloan EK, Capitanio JP, Cole SW: Stress-induced remodeling of lymphoid innervation. Brain Behav Immun 22(1):15–21, 2008 17697764

Stein JY, Levin Y, Uziel O, et al: Traumatic stress and cellular senescence: the role of war-captivity and homecoming stressors in later life telomere length. J Affect Disord 238:129–135, 2018 29879607

Steptoe A, Owen N, Kunz-Ebrecht SR, Brydon L: Loneliness and neuroendocrine, cardiovascular, and inflammatory stress responses in middle-aged men and women. Psychoneuroendocrinology 29(5):593–611, 2004 15041083

Theeke LA, Mallow JA, Moore J, et al: Using gene expression analysis to examine changes in loneliness, depression and systemic inflammation in lonely chronically ill older adults. Open J Nurs 6(8):620–631, 2016 29082106

Vingeliene S, Hiyoshi A, Lentjes M, et al: Longitudinal analysis of loneliness and inflammation at older ages: English longitudinal study of ageing. Psychoneuroendocrinology 110:104421, 2019 31494341

Walker E, Ploubidis G, Fancourt D: Social engagement and loneliness are differentially associated with neuro-immune markers in older age: time-varying associations from the English Longitudinal Study of Ageing. Brain Behav Immun 82:224–229, 2019 31491488

Wohleb ES, McKim DB, Sheridan JF, Godbout JP: Monocyte trafficking to the brain with stress and inflammation: a novel axis of immune-to-brain communication that influences mood and behavior. Front Neurosci 9:447, 2015 25653581

Zilioli S, Slatcher RB, Chi P, et al: The impact of daily and trait loneliness on diurnal cortisol and sleep among children affected by parental HIV/AIDS. Psychoneuroendocrinology 75:64–71, 2017 27810705

Interventions for Loneliness in Younger People

Pamela Qualter, Ph.D.
Alice Eccles, Ph.D.
Manuela Barreto, Ph.D.

Loneliness Among Young People

Loneliness among school-age children and adolescents is a painful experience associated with feeling unhappy, unloved, restless, and despondent (Yang et al. 2022). It is related to the absence of play partners during childhood and a lack of close friends during adolescence (Qualter et al. 2015). Loneliness is not just about the absence of positive social relationships, however; it can also be linked to the presence of negative social relationships, including victimization (Kochenderfer-Ladd and Wardrop 2001; Matthews

The authors would like to thank Margaret Duncan, M.D., for contributing the case vignette.

et al. 2022; Yang et al. 2022) and peer group rejection (Matthews et al. 2019a; Qualter and Munn 2002; Qualter et al. 2015).

The negative emotions experienced when people are lonely are thought to motivate them to overcome loneliness (see Chapter 2, "Loneliness, Other Aspects of Social Connection, and Their Measurement"), and that is the case across the life span (Qualter et al. 2015). To overcome those uncomfortable negative emotions, we are motivated to reconnect with others and to renew social connections. Most people do reconnect, but when loneliness continues for some time during childhood and adolescence, it increases the risk of depression and anxiety (for a review, see Loades et al. 2020), engagement in self-harm behavior (Yang et al. 2022), poor reported physical health (Christiansen et al. 2021), and poor sleep (Harris et al. 2013; Matthews et al. 2017). The impacts also go beyond health: loneliness is associated with poor academic performance (Eccles and Qualter 2021; Qualter et al. 2021a) and, in late adolescence and emerging adulthood, is linked to job-seeking struggles (Matthews et al. 2019a).

Recent research has drawn attention to the presence and prevalence of loneliness in adolescence and young adulthood (Barreto et al. 2021c; Luhmann and Hawkley 2016; Office for National Statistics 2018), with data from national surveys showing that about 10% of 16- to 24-year-olds report loneliness "often" or "always" compared with an average of 5% for other age groups. There have been few population-based surveys of loneliness among younger adolescents, and those available suggest that between 6% and 8% of adolescents ages 11–15 years felt loneliness "always" or "often" (Qualter et al. 2021a; see also Madsen et al. 2019; Yang et al. 2022). Research has noted an increase in loneliness for adolescents in Denmark from 1995 to 2014 (Madsen et al. 2019), although it remained lower for the United Kingdom over that period (Qualter et al. 2021a). In the United Kingdom, loneliness was stable for those ages 13–15 years from 2006 to 2014 and decreased for 11-year-olds between 2002 and 2014 (Qualter et al. 2021a). There are no data for recent years available from adolescents younger than 16. There are also no population-based surveys of loneliness among children younger than 11, so there are no prevalence data available for children.

Measuring Youth Loneliness

A recent review (Cole et al. 2021) assessed the psychometric properties of the three most popular measures of loneliness for youth—UCLA Loneliness Scale (UCLA LS; Russell et al. 1978), Children's Loneliness and Social Dissatisfaction Scale (CLS; Asher et al. 1984), and Loneliness and Aloneness Scale for Children and Adolescents (LACA; Marcoen et al. 1987). The review showed that versions of the UCLA LS are the most popular for examining loneliness among adolescents, although few studies note its psychometric properties when used with that age group; for children, the CLS was the most suitable. The authors identified important gaps in aspects of measure development, with no measure for youth having been developed with children or adolescents (Cole et al. 2021).

Single-item measures of loneliness have also been used with different age groups. In one study with 11- to 15-year-olds (Eccles et al. 2020), a single-item loneliness measure that asked, "Do you feel lonely?" was compared with the four-item UCLA measure (Roberts et al. 1993). The findings showed that the two measures were highly correlated but that adolescents who were identified as lonely using one measurement of loneliness were not always identified as such on the other measure. That finding is consistent with evidence from comparison of direct and indirect measures of loneliness among adults (Shiovitz-Ezra and Ayalon 2012; Victor et al. 2005). Fewer people identify as "lonely" using direct measures of loneliness than when a composite measure is used that does not use the word *lonely*, likely related to the stigma surrounding loneliness that is evident across the life span (Barreto et al. 2021b).

Despite the limitations of direct measures of loneliness, one advantage is that they include a specific time frame (e.g., 1 week) for reference, something that is not included in composite loneliness measures such as the UCLA scale. Indirect composite measures of loneliness ask about the relative frequency with which one experiences loneliness (hardly ever, some of the time, often) but not a specific time frame, such as every day, half the days, or every few days (Qualter et al. 2021b). These reference points are considered important in the clinical examination of depression (Krabbe and Forkmann 2012) because they enable participants to provide greater accuracy regarding the frequency of their experiences. Specific time frames are currently missing from loneliness measures other than the single-item questions.

An issue for loneliness measures in general, and not one restricted to measures for youth, is that there are no known predetermined cutoffs indicating difficulties. Thus, there is no standardized way to identify those children and adolescents reporting loneliness who need extra support. That said, those who report feeling lonely all or almost all of the time have been shown to have different behavioral and cognitive profiles from the remainder of each sample (Adams et al. 2004; Bangee et al. 2014; Qualter et al. 2013b), suggesting such a cutoff could be used to identify those most in need of intervention.

Risk Factors for Loneliness

Research has demonstrated that risk factors for youth loneliness exist at multiple levels, including individual factors, aspects of interpersonal relationships, characteristics of the individual's living situation (which we refer to as *situational*), sociocultural factors, and demographics (Table 8–1). These factors often co-occur and are interrelated, also within levels of analysis.

Individual Factors

Attitude Toward Being Alone

Spending a lot of time alone is a risk factor for youth loneliness, especially if it is a result of lack of access to people with whom to socialize (Maes et al. 2016). Although spending time alone can also be important for young people if it is used for self-developmental purposes (Long and Averill 2003), it seems to be linked to loneliness when aloneness is not a choice (Vanhalst et al. 2013a, 2013b). At the same time, positive attitudes toward aloneness can lead to exaggerated time alone ("too much of a good thing"), which can lead to loneliness (Wang et al. 2013).

Personality

High introversion, low agreeableness, low conscientiousness, and high neuroticism influence attitudes about being alone, social avoidance, and social behavior in social interactions, which in turn influence loneliness (Bueckner et al. 2020). Differences in introversion can be particularly important in relationship initiation, with neuroticism, agreeableness, and conscientiousness being stronger predictors of later relationship quality (Klimstra et al. 2013).

Poor or Atypical Social Skills

Individual differences in social skills, such as assertion, cooperation, interpersonal empathy, peer competence, and self-control in social interactions can predict loneliness in children and young people (Schinka et al. 2013). Some researchers have proposed that poor social skills explain a high prevalence of loneliness in autistic individuals (e.g., Lasgaard et al. 2010), but others have pointed out that it might be more helpful to regard these skills as *atypical* rather than deficient. Indeed, autistic children are very able to establish close relationships that are mutually satisfying for them and their friends (Petrina et al. 2017). However, their atypical social skills can clash with those of neurotypical children, which leads to difficulties in interactions with those who are not yet close and, therefore, this presents a risk for loneliness in this group.

Maladaptive Cognitions

Those who report loneliness frequently have been found to engage in cognitions that both predispose them to loneliness and make it hard to over-

TABLE 8–1.   **Risk factors associated with youth loneliness and how those are, and could be, addressed by interventions**

Risk factors	Interventions that address risk factors
Individual	**Existing interventions**
Attitude toward being alone	Social skills training
Personality (especially introversion)	Socioemotional skills training
Identity change	Psychological therapies
Poor or atypical social skills	
Unhelpful cognitions	
Affectivity and emotion regulation	
Mental ill health	
Physical ill health and disability	
Interpersonal	**Existing interventions**
Quantity of friends	Increasing social interaction opportunities
Poor quality friendships	Social skills training
Peer victimization	Socioemotional skills training
	Psychological therapies
Situational	**Existing interventions**
Social isolation	Enhanced social support
Life transitions	**Interventions that could address risk factors***
Adversity	
Social media use	Improve transportation
	Provide support around life transitions
	Support sensible internet use
Sociocultural	**Potential interventions***
Neighborhood characteristics	Improve housing so people can live in nice neighborhoods and closer to towns
Cultural individualism	Improve meeting spaces in residential areas
Cultural prejudice	Improve community cohesion and involvement in neighborhood decisions
	Promote inclusive environments (in and outside of school), including teaching youth to use basic sign language, understanding of different needs, and communication strategies

TABLE 8–1. Risk factors associated with youth loneliness and how those are, and could be, addressed by interventions *(continued)*

Risk factors	Interventions that address risk factors
Demographic	
Sex/Gender	
Education level	
Unemployment	

Note. *Where no existing interventions are available.

come lonely feelings. For example, individuals who feel lonely are prone to attribute social exclusion to their personal characteristics (e.g., Qualter et al. 2013a; Renshaw and Brown 1993), while attributing inclusion to circumstances (Qualter and Munn 2002; Vanhalst et al. 2015). They also tend to perceive that they have no control over whether they are included (Jones et al. 1981). Youth who frequently feel lonely have also been shown to have negative views of others, seeing others as less trustworthy, less supportive, and less socially desirable (Jones et al. 1981; Qualter et al. 2013a; Rotenberg et al. 2010). People who often feel lonely also display increased vigilance for social threats (Bangee et al. 2014; Masi et al. 2011) and tend to fear and expect that others will reject them (Jackson 2007; Qualter et al. 2013b).

Affectivity and Emotion Regulation

Adolescents who report feeling lonely often have an impaired ability to enjoy inclusion and show more negative affective responses to exclusion than adolescents who do not report feeling lonely (Vanhalst et al. 2015). Furthermore, evidence suggests that youth who experience persistent loneliness have heightened emotional intensity for both positive and negative emotions (Davis et al. 2019). In addition, low self-esteem is consistently associated with loneliness, with the relationship being bidirectional: low self-esteem causes loneliness, which in turn decreases self-esteem (Vanhalst et al. 2013a, 2013b). We can see how low self-esteem, particularly when combined with negative cognitions, provides a foundation for the belief that loneliness cannot be remedied (Qualter et al. 2015).

Poor Mental Health

In addition to negatively affecting mental health (Loades et al. 2020), loneliness can emerge from poor mental health (Lasgaard et al. 2016). For example, loneliness is both a driver of and aggravated by eating disorders (Levine 2012), and it can become more severe during the course of a mental illness

(Wang et al. 2020). Childhood experiences of mental illness not only shape loneliness when they happen but also shape loneliness in later life (Matthews et al. 2019a, 2019b). Such effects are partly due to the direct effects of symptoms of the illness itself (e.g., reduced energy or confidence) on social interactions, but social stigma and discrimination also play an important role.

The relationship between mental illness and loneliness depends on the specific mental illness, with individuals with psychotic disorders not showing that relationship to the same extent as individuals with mood or personality disorders (Alasmawi et al. 2020). In addition, different types of mental health issues can be associated with different types of social difficulties. For example, peer- and family-related (but not romantic) loneliness have been associated with anxiety, depression, and suicide ideation in high school students; peer and romantic (but not family) loneliness were associated with social phobia; and family (but not peer or romantic) loneliness was related to self-harm and eating disorders (Lasgaard et al. 2011).

Poor Physical Health and Disability

Young people with a chronic physical illness (Jeon et al. 2010) or a physical disability (Tough et al. 2017) report significant loneliness. This can be associated with obstacles to social participation that are related to the condition (e.g., reduced mobility, reduced energy levels, pain, or socially unacceptable symptoms) and to external barriers such as stigma and the lack of accessible social spaces. Children with visual or hearing impairments are specifically affected due to how the impairment affects their communication with non-impaired children (Maes et al. 2017) and the latter's lack of skills to interact with impaired children (e.g., not knowing sign language).

Interpersonal Factors

Number of Friends

In the earliest stages of life, social relationships are often restricted to parents and other family members, and friendships with peers are mainly defined by the availability of peers with whom to share activities, such as playing. Not having peers to play with is, thus, an important driver of loneliness in young children (Renshaw and Brown 1993). Whether young people are likely to be happy with their social connections also depends on how they perceive those connections to measure up to the connections they believe their peers have (Laursen and Hartl 2013). This can lead to unrealistic standards because young people often overestimate how many friends others have (Deri et al. 2017), something to which social media greatly contributes (Lee 2014). Indeed, the value of social connection is so high that people often go out of their way to present themselves as well connected, especially on social media (Zhao et al. 2008).

Poor Relationship Quality

As children grow, they become preoccupied with being accepted by their peer group. In this developmental process, a lack of peer acceptance is a significant predictor of loneliness (Vanhalst et al. 2014), and positive peer functioning is a key predictor of low loneliness across childhood (Jobe-Shields et al. 2011). Throughout adolescence and emerging adulthood, romantic relationships become important too, and a lack thereof becomes an important determinant of loneliness (Qualter et al. 2015).

Peer Victimization

Various forms of social victimization (e.g., ostracism, exclusion, bullying) predict loneliness across childhood (Kochenderfer-Ladd and Wardrop 2001), adolescence (Yang et al. 2022), and emerging adulthood (Matthews et al. 2022). In fact, early experiences with victimization have been found to predict loneliness not only when the victimization occurs but also later in life (Matthews et al. 2022). Victimization directly affects social networks and affects youths' psychological makeup in ways that impede positive relationships (e.g., decreasing self-esteem and increasing social anxiety and rejection sensitivity) (Iffland et al. 2014; Zimmer-Gembeck et al. 2014).

Situational Factors

Social Isolation

The young person's life circumstances also constitute risk factors for loneliness. Living alone, for example, has been found to predict severe loneliness across the life span (Lasgaard et al. 2016). Adolescents are particularly averse to spending a lot of time alone, although they sometimes feel less lonely alone than in the company of others who are not their friends (van Roekel et al. 2015). Another source of social isolation is living in remote rural areas, which reduces social opportunities and increases difficulties accessing places where social events take place. Indeed, young people living in rural areas have been shown to report more loneliness than those living in cities (Chipuer and Pretty 2000).

Life Transitions

Young people often undergo significant life transitions, such as moving or changing schools, and those go hand in hand with changes in social networks, which can increase loneliness (Ladd and Ettekal 2013). An important life transition for young people is moving away from home for the first time, for example, the transition to university, which has been associated with heightened levels of loneliness as young people adjust to this new life (Nightingale et al. 2013). Youth with disabilities are particularly vulnerable to loneliness after leaving school as they encounter barriers to further education or employment that leave them feeling left out (Ravenscroft et al. 2017).

Other important life transitions and drivers of loneliness relate to identity exploration, development, and change. Although these are normal developmental processes in adolescence and emerging adulthood, at times they can be associated with conflict with friends and family, such as when new values or activities are incompatible with old ones (Laursen and Hartl 2013). Identity development can be associated with loneliness particularly when it is accompanied by poor self-acceptance (or self-stigma), lack of identity clarity, or prejudice and discrimination. For example, the development of a sexual minority identity (Halpin and Allen 2004) and of a transgender identity (Levitt and Ippolito 2014) can both be associated with loneliness until a stage of acceptance is reached.

Adverse Life Experiences

Adverse life experiences can impact/contribute to loneliness both when they happen and later on in life. For example, poverty (Qualter et al. 2021a) and homelessness (Kidd 2007) have been associated with high levels of loneliness in young people, whereas high family income predicted stable low levels of loneliness across childhood (Schinka et al. 2013). Physical, emotional, and sexual abuse in childhood have also been linked to loneliness in emerging adulthood (Lev-Wiesel and Sternberg 2012) and later (Merz and Jak 2013).

Social Media Use

Social media limits time spent in face-to-face interactions and can encourage the development of unrealistic social standards. Young people spend most of their time on social media viewing other people's profiles (Pempek et al. 2009), and most social comparisons on social media are upward comparisons that can leave young people feeling inferior and left out (Vogel et al. 2015). One study experimentally demonstrated that Facebook use increased both depression and loneliness (Hunt et al. 2018). However, in a review of the literature, Nowland et al. (2018) argued that young people who use social media can benefit if social media is used to extend face-to-face social interactions rather than to replace them. Still, even when social media is used to replace face-to-face social interactions, it might prevent loneliness if other opportunities for social interactions are truly limited (e.g., due to lack of access to relevant others). Social media can also be an important source of connection during life transitions, enabling young people to retain connections they already had or to explore new connections (Thomas et al. 2020).

Sociocultural Factors

Neighborhood Characteristics

Neighborhood deprivation, lack of resources, poor social capital, and local norms regarding helpfulness and friendliness have been shown to influence children and adolescent health and well-being (Kearns et al. 2015; Leventhal and Brooks-Gunn 2000). For example, positive and trusting relationships with neighbors and perceived neighborhood cohesion can benefit mental health and protect against loneliness (Matthews et al. 2019b). Characteristics of the built environment (e.g., lack of social spaces, degradation, lack of safety) and poor transportation can also limit opportunities for social interaction (Mazumdar et al. 2018), but their impact specifically on young populations has not yet been well researched.

Cultural Individualism

Evidence for how cultural individualism affects young people's feelings of loneliness is scarce and somewhat inconsistent. Although there is evidence that young people feel lonelier in collectivist societies (Lykes and Kemmelmeier 2014), evidence also shows that they feel lonelier in individualistic societies (Barreto et al. 2021c). Heu et al. (2019) showed that cultural individualism does not shape standards for connection but reduces the extent to which individuals are actually connected. It also seems that culture influences what aspects of social life drive feelings of loneliness: Having a close confidant is a stronger determinant of loneliness in individualistic societies than it is in collectivist societies (Lykes and Kemmelmeier 2014). At the same time, young people living in collectivist societies are more likely to blame themselves for disconnection than are young people in individualistic societies (Anderson 1999; Barreto et al. 2021c), suggesting that loneliness might be more impactful for those living in collectivist environments. Furthermore, research shows that individuals living in collectivist environments are protected from rare negative social experiences but are generally more fearful of exclusion than people living in individualistic societies (Uskul and Over 2017).

Cultural Prejudice

Research has highlighted disparities in the extent to which members of different minority and majority groups in society experience loneliness. For example, studies have demonstrated that ethnic minority status is associated with increased loneliness in all age groups (e.g., Lasgaard et al. 2016); young migrants report more loneliness than those without a migration experience (Madsen et al. 2016); and sexual minority individuals report more loneliness than heterosexual persons (Doyle and Molix 2016). Multiple studies suggest that these discrepancies might be related to differential exposure to harassment and discrimination (Barreto et al. 2021a; Doyle and Barreto 2021; Priest et al. 2017). Experiences with discrimination can affect the quantity and quality of social relationships by 1) excluding minority individuals from social networks and 2) affecting their affect and cognition in ways that impair satisfactory social engagement. Cultural prejudice might also contribute to the risk associated with factors discussed in other sections, such as disability or low socioeconomic status.

Demographic Factors

A range of demographic factors have been associated with loneliness, with effects often determined by developmental, individual, or sociocultural factors. For example, low education level (Lasgaard et al. 2016) and unemployment (Matthews et al. 2019a) are associated with loneliness in emerging adults. Such variables can determine whether young people have the financial resources so often required to participate in social events, but they can also go hand in hand with low self-esteem, neighborhood deprivation, and cultural prejudice.

Although studies frequently report sex effects, a recent meta-analysis revealed that the effects of sex on loneliness across the life span are negligible (Maes et al. 2019). Others have found that effects of sex depend on whether the questions used to assess loneliness directly ask about feelings of loneliness (Borys and Perlman 1985), because men (of all ages) are more likely to perceive a stigma associated with feeling lonely (Barreto et al. 2021a). (Please see Chapter 3, "Loneliness Across the Life Span," for related information.)

Interventions Aimed at Alleviating Youth Loneliness

To date, only one meta-analytical study has been published examining the effectiveness of interventions used for alleviating loneliness in young people (Eccles and Qualter 2021). That meta-analysis included 39 studies (14 single-group design and 25 randomized controlled trials [RCTs]) that focused exclusively on young people ages 3–25 years. The review examined the effectiveness of interventions and the role of important, theoretically driven moderators, including intervention focus, delivery format, and sample demographics. The results suggest that interventions are moderately effective at alleviating loneliness, with an effect size of 0.316 for RCTs and 0.411 for pre/post intervention studies. Since publication of that meta-analysis, only one pre/post intervention study has been done (Agadullina et al. 2020) that would meet its inclusion criteria.

Interventions in Relation to Identified Risk Factors

The loneliness interventions currently available for youth have focused on different risk factors. For example, some interventions target social isolation, whereas others focus on addressing the maladaptive cognitions that accompany loneliness. Table 8–2 highlights the different foci of the current interventions, mapped onto the following risk factors for loneliness among youth: 1) individual differences, 2) interpersonal, 3) situational, and 4) sociocultural. Table 8–2 also notes the papers in which interventions have been evaluated and where further details can be found. It is clear from the table that most interventions have focused on individual differences, interpersonal, and situational factors. Only one has focused on sociocultural risk factors, and it is important to note that this intervention was focused on how individuals manage cultural prejudice rather than on targeted change within the system.

Individual Differences

Most of the interventions in Table 8–2 address risk factors at the individual differences level. There are interventions designed for young people with autism spectrum disorder (ASD), social phobia, behavioral problems, and higher reports of loneliness or depression. Most interventions focus on the development of emotional or social skills, with the aim of improving interaction with peers. Other interventions offer psychological therapies that aim to modify maladaptive cognitions and enable adoption of adaptive coping strategies.

Eccles and Qualter (2021) showed that interventions aimed at specific individual risk factors are not consistently successful. For example, for those studies that included young people with ASD, interventions aimed to develop socioemotional skills reported a significant reduction in reports of loneliness in some studies (Bradley 2016; Frankel et al. 2010; Gantman et al. 2012) but not others (Barry et al. 2003; Deckers et al. 2016). Research has started to show how particular environments can facilitate interactions with and between autistic individuals, reducing feelings of loneliness (Kim and

TABLE 8–2. An overview of studies included in the Eccles and Qualter (2021) review including target sample, intervention focus, and associated risk factors

Intervention studies of related risk factors and intervention focus*	Summary of sample (age range, years)	Brief description of intervention
Individual differences		
Social skills training		
Margalit 1995b	Students with special needs, including learning disabilities and behavioral disorders (11–15)	I Found A Solution: Computer-based program that includes interpersonal conflict scenarios and adventure games to reflect difficult social events.
Beidel et al. 2000	School-age children with social phobia (8–12)	Social Effectiveness Therapy for Children: A multifaceted behavioral treatment model to address various dimensions of social anxiety including reduction in fear, improvement in social skills, and increase in participation of social activities.
Barry et al. 2003	High-functioning school children with ASD (6–9)	Designed to teach specific social skills (including greetings and conversations) through eight group sessions.
Masia-Warner et al. 2005	Adolescents with a specific subtype of social phobia or social anxiety disorder (13–17)	Skills for Social and Academic Success: Intervention includes sessions focused on the modification and implementation of social skills in a relevant setting (i.e., school environment).
Frankel et al. 2010	Children who satisfied ASD criteria (7–11)	Children's Friendship Training: A program teaching social etiquette and social skills. Skills include conversational skills, developing friendships, and good sportsmanship.

TABLE 8–2. An overview of studies included in the Eccles and Qualter (2021) review including target sample, intervention focus, and associated risk factors *(continued)*

Intervention studies of related risk factors and intervention focus*	Summary of sample (age range, years)	Brief description of intervention
Individual differences *(continued)*		
Social skills training (continued)		
Gantman et al. 2012	Young adults with ASD (18–23)	UCLA PEERS for young adults: Community-delivered intervention focused on building close relationships and on skills such as communication, conversation, and handling social situations.
Social and emotional skills		
Bostick and Anderson 2009	School children identified as needing counseling according to scores on loneliness and social anxiety measures (8–9)	S.S. Grin: Structured, cognitive behavioral intervention with detailed scripts and activities. Intervention focuses on verbal and nonverbal communication, initiations, cooperation, negotiation skills, emotional regulation, and perspective taking.
Craig et al. 2016	School-age children with access to the internet (7–11)	Zoo-U: Technology-based social skills training program that uses adaptive scenes to identify strengths and weaknesses in social skill set. Focuses on six core skills, including social literary, self-efficacy, and peer relations.
Deckers et al. 2016	Children with a formal diagnosis of pervasive developmental disorder not otherwise specified, Asperger's disorder, or autistic disorder (8–12)	Group intervention focusing on basic social skills training (including eye contact and voice volume) and turn-taking. More advanced social skills also included in the intervention, including listening, emotion recognition, and saying no.

TABLE 8–2. An overview of studies included in the Eccles and Qualter (2021) review including target sample, intervention focus, and associated risk factors *(continued)*

Intervention studies of related risk factors and intervention focus*	Summary of sample (age range, years)	Brief description of intervention
Individual differences (continued)		
Social and emotional skills (continued)		
Margalit 1995a	Children with mild intellectual disability (11–15)	I Found A Solution: Computer-based program that includes interpersonal conflict scenarios and adventure games to reflect difficult social events and related emotions.
Leff et al. 2009	Relationally aggressive girls (8–12)	Friend2Friend: Developed specifically to focus on aggression among girls. Program includes components focused on friendship problems, coping strategies, evaluation of intentions/responses, and application of strategies to peer interactions.
Kjøbli and Ogden 2014	Children who displayed problem behaviors (e.g., aggression, delinquency) at day care or at school (3–12)	Individual social skills training: Intervention aimed at improving social skills and emotional regulation. Also focuses on coping mechanisms for maladaptive behavior and problem-solving.
Sanchez et al. 2017	School children identified as "at risk" on the behavior assessment system for children (7–11)	Adventures: Adventure-based intervention focusing on social and emotional skills.

TABLE 8–2. An overview of studies included in the Eccles and Qualter (2021) review including target sample, intervention focus, and associated risk factors (*continued*)

Intervention studies of related risk factors and intervention focus*	Summary of sample (age range, years)	Brief description of intervention
Individual differences (*continued*)		
Psychological intervention		
Klingman and Hochdorf 1993	School-age children (12.5–13.5)	Intervention based on rational emotive education and cognitive modifications.
Stice et al. 2010	At-risk teens with elevated depressive symptoms (14–19)	Cognitive-behavioral depression prevention program delivered over five steps.
Diab et al. 2014	War-affected children (10–13)	Teaching recovery techniques focusing on psychoeducation and cognitive-behavioral therapy linked to trauma. Trains effective coping skills and regulation of emotions and facilitates integrating overwhelming traumatic memories.
Brouzos et al. 2016	School children wearing glasses (9–12)	Storytelling intervention group designed to increase emotional wellness and decrease levels of social anxiety/shyness. Designed to help children alter the way they perceive social interaction, discuss emotions, and explore issues faced by individuals with low vision.
Mason et al. 2016	Adolescents at high risk of substance abuse and presenting at a primary care clinic (14–18)	Peer network counseling: Focuses on rapport building, discussion of substance use, peer networks, and behavioral modification.

TABLE 8–2. An overview of studies included in the Eccles and Qualter (2021) review including target sample, intervention focus, and associated risk factors *(continued)*

Intervention studies of related risk factors and intervention focus*	Summary of sample (age range, years)	Brief description of intervention
Individual differences *(continued)*		
Psychological intervention (continued)		
Zhang et al. 2016	Chinese college students with elevated loneliness (17–25)	Mindfulness-based cognitive therapy aimed at increasing moment-by-moment awareness and addressing maladaptive thought processes.
Vassilopoulos et al. 2018	Adolescents enrolled in Year 6 of Greek school (11–12)	A short, problem-oriented group program focused on interpretation retraining, problem solving, and social skills development.
Learning new skills		
Regev and Guttmann 2005	Primary school children with learning disorders (8.5–13)	Experimental art group to ease personal difficulties and encourage personal identity growth.
Interpersonal factors		
Increasing social interaction		
Battles and Wiener 2002	Young patients with potentially life-threatening illnesses (including HIV) (8–19)	STARBRIGHT World: Electronic network designed for children/adolescents with prolonged illness or injury. Intervention addresses the psychosocial challenges that arise from being "inhibited from normal play."

TABLE 8–2. An overview of studies included in the Eccles and Qualter (2021) review including target sample, intervention focus, and associated risk factors (*continued*)

Intervention studies of related risk factors and intervention focus*	Summary of sample (age range, *years*)	Brief description of intervention
Interpersonal factors (*continued*)		
Increasing social interaction (*continued*)		
Grace et al. 2014	Young people with complex communication needs because of physical disability, condition, or acquired brain injury (10–15)	Intervention program to increase social connection. Includes provision of technological solutions, support, and training to overcome opportunity and access barriers to internet use to encourage independence to access emails and video calling as well as accessibility technologies.
Lim et al. 2019	Adolescents with a social anxiety disorder (18–24)	+Connect: Smart phone intervention that uses videos/daily posts to strengthen relationships and increase social connection.
Social skills training		
King et al. 1997	Children with a diagnosis of cerebral palsy or spina bifida. Problems with peer relations (8–15)	Joining In: Program designed to address neurocognitive, social, and physical characteristics of children with physical disabilities. Sessions focused on interpersonal problem solving, verbal and nonverbal communication, initiating interactions with peers, conversational skills, and coping with difficult others.

TABLE 8–2. An overview of studies included in the Eccles and Qualter (2021) review including target sample, intervention focus, and associated risk factors (*continued*)

Intervention studies of related risk factors and intervention focus*	Summary of sample (age range, years)	Brief description of intervention
Interpersonal factors (*continued*)		
Social and emotional skills		
Christian and D'Auria 2006	School-age children with cystic fibrosis (8–12)	Building Life Skills: Social and emotional skills intervention to deal with specific problems ranging from finding out about diagnoses to keeping up with peers during physical activities.
Cross et al. 2018	Adolescents enrolled in Grades 7 and 8 (12–14)	Friendly School Project: Focused on reducing bullying and encouraging students' normative beliefs about non-acceptance of bullying. Intervention aims to increase feelings of support, improve empathy and social competence, increase feelings of school-connectedness, and reduce self-reported loneliness.
Other		
Kopelman-Rubin et al. 2012	Young adolescents with learning disorders (11–15)	"I Can Succeed": Aims to promote academic and emotional function of adolescents and focuses on intrapersonal, interpersonal, and school/community level goals. Focuses on relationship between family and school, individual and family, and individual and school.

TABLE 8–2. An overview of studies included in the Eccles and Qualter (2021) review including target sample, intervention focus, and associated risk factors (*continued*)

Intervention studies of related risk factors and intervention focus*	Summary of sample (age range, years)	Brief description of intervention
Situation factors		
Enhancing social support		
Mattanah et al. 2010	First-year college students (17–19)	Group-based intervention to ease transition into new educational setting. Sessions facilitated by older students and include topics such as creating new social ties, balancing life and study commitments, and expectations of college life.
Stewart et al. 2011	Children with physical disabilities including cerebral palsy and spina bifida (12–18)	Ability Online: Integrated platform for email, message board, and chat rooms.
Stewart et al. 2013	Children with either allergies, asthma, or both (7–11)	GoToMeeting and Club Penguin: Online platforms to encourage group support and social interactions.
Bradley 2016	School children with ASD (11–12)	Peer mentoring program designed to provide a safe space to discuss and problem-solve issues, including friendships, bullying, interests, and behavior.
Matthews et al. 2018	Adolescents diagnosed with ASD (13–17)	PEERS with peers: Peer-mediated intervention with strategies relating to proximity and initiation.

TABLE 8–2. An overview of studies included in the Eccles and Qualter (2021) review including target sample, intervention focus, and associated risk factors *(continued)*

Intervention studies of related risk factors and intervention focus*	Summary of sample (age range, *years*)	Brief description of intervention
Situation factors *(continued)*		
Enhancing social support (continued)		
Kneer et al. 2019	Migrant youth (13–18)	Peer2Peer: Method of coaching aimed to make adolescents more successful in their school career. Through a peers and buddy system, the program helps to develop skills relating to reflection and teamwork.
Larsen et al. 2019	Adolescents enrolled in upper secondary school (15–19)	Dream School Program: Whole-school initiative to help encourage a sense of belonging and promote mental health. Uses a peer leader system.
Psychological intervention		
Quayle et al. 2001	Girls about to transition to high school (11–12)	Optimism and Lifeskills Program: Encourages pupils to challenge negative thoughts and encourages adaptive coping strategies.
Rohde et al. 2004	Incarcerated young males (12–22)	Coping Course: Aimed at improving social skills, cognitive reconstruction, and coping mechanisms with mood. Modified for current sample to focus on coping with negative emotions such as sadness, fear, and boredom.

TABLE 8–2. An overview of studies included in the Eccles and Qualter (2021) review including target sample, intervention focus, and associated risk factors (*continued*)

Intervention studies of related risk factors and intervention focus*	Summary of sample (age range, years)	Brief description of intervention
Situation factors (*continued*)		
Sensible media use		
Agadullina et al. 2020**	First-year university students (mean 19.9)	Includes quitting social network sites for 4 weeks.
Learning new skills		
Purohit et al. 2016	Orphaned adolescents (11–16)	Practical, yoga-based intervention program.
Sociocultural factors		
Psychological intervention		
Smith et al. 2017	Gay and bisexual young males (18–25)	Project PRIDE: Group intervention focusing on coping strategies (including maladaptive) and goal setting.

Note. ASD=autism spectrum disorder.
*Intervention focus as classified in Eccles and Qualter (2021).
**Published after the Eccles and Qualter meta-analysis but fits criteria.

Bottema-Beutel 2019; Sosnowy et al. 2018), and such work could be used to inform current and future interventions for those with ASD who report loneliness.

Psychological therapy aimed at reducing maladaptive cognitions and increasing adaptive coping strategies among youth seem to be effective in all available studies (Brouzos et al. 2016; Stice et al. 2010; Zhang et al. 2016). For example, Zhang et al. (2016) used mindfulness-based cognitive therapy to help address maladaptive thought processes in college students with elevated reports of loneliness and showed a significant reduction in loneliness. Using cognitive-behavioral therapy, Stice et al. (2010) reported a significant reduction in loneliness in at-risk teens with elevated depressive symptoms. Brouzos et al. (2016) reported a significant reduction in loneliness in school-age children who wore glasses following a 6-week storytelling intervention. Thus, interventions focusing on changing and altering maladaptive cognitive biases might offer an effective intervention therapy for youth reporting loneliness.

Interpersonal Factors

Many of the interventions aimed at improving interpersonal relationships focus on increasing peer interactions, developing emotional or social skills, and enhancing social support. They are aimed at children and adolescents with long-term health conditions that act as barriers to normative play and interpersonal interactions.

Most interventions that address interpersonal factors report nonsignificant reductions in loneliness. However, two studies report a significant reduction in loneliness pre- and post-intervention (Battles and Wiener 2002; Cross et al. 2018). Cross et al. (2018) described a school-wide initiative focusing on social and emotional skills aimed at reducing bullying, encouraging positive social relations, and developing school-connectedness across all students. This approach addressed certain risk factors we identify as sociocultural to create an inclusive school climate. Battles and Wiener (2002) examined STARBRIGHT, a technology-based intervention that addresses the psychosocial challenges that arise for inhibited normative play for young patients with potentially life-threatening diseases by increasing their opportunities for social interactions. STARBRIGHT is an electronic network providing an interactive community for children and adolescents with serious illnesses. Findings from Battles and Weiner suggest that STARBRIGHT provided a sense of connectedness for children who could otherwise feel isolated from their peers. Furthermore, results suggest that although children did not spend excessive amounts of time online, the idea that "simply knowing that other children similar to themselves are out there" (p. 62) may have been enough to reduce feelings of loneliness.

Situational Factors

Most interventions that aim to address situational risk factors focus on enhancing social support and social isolation during life transitions. Initiatives mainly encourage engagement with peers having a similar experience. Mattanah et al. (2010) evaluated one such intervention. They reported a significant reduction in feelings of loneliness among first-year college students who met with older students and discussed topics relating to new and old social relationships, balancing life and study commitments, and setting expectations of college life. Although this study showed the intervention to be successful at reducing loneliness, not all interventions to enhance social support have been as successful; these include interventions using coaching (Kneer et al. 2019), peer mentoring (Bradley 2016), and peer-leader-based support systems (Larsen et al. 2019). There are also interventions designed for youth in specific contexts, such as those in incarceration (Rohde et al. 2004) and those experiencing school transition (Quayle et al. 2001), for whom there is increased risk of loneliness. Other interventions address situational risk for loneliness through teaching new skills and encouraging effective coping (Purohit et al. 2016). However, these studies did not report a significant reduction in loneliness. Findings from those interventions focusing on situational factors have been mixed and, therefore, highlight the importance of considering the underlying risk factors when designing a targeted intervention to alleviate loneliness.

Sociocultural Factors

Currently, only one intervention has been empirically evaluated that could be classified as targeting cultural prejudice. Smith et al. (2017) reported significant yet small reductions in loneliness pre- and post-intervention in a sample of gay and bisexual men ages 18–25 years. The PRIDE intervention includes eight sessions focused on different aspects, including psychoeducation, modeling and roleplaying sexual communication skills, and emotion- and problem-focused coping strategies. PRIDE has elements of homework and target setting to encourage engagement and application of newly acquired skills and knowledge. Although the results of the study look promising, this intervention focuses on those at risk for the negative experience of stigma and alienation. Future interventions addressing sociocultural risk factors should also consider whether the promotion of inclusion and improvement in community cohesion can address this risk factor more effectively.

Evaluation of Youth Interventions and Recommendations for Future Work

In their evaluation of the currently available, empirically evaluated interventions, Eccles and Qualter (2021) showed that many evaluation studies did not specifically target young people who reported loneliness. Those that did target youth who frequently experienced loneliness showed reductions in loneliness. However, instead of focusing the intervention on youth reporting frequent loneliness, interventions often were evaluated with youth from populations that the adults thought would be lonely (i.e., at-risk samples). That means some of the interventions for which no reductions in loneliness were detected by the study teams might have been more effective if the targeted samples had actually reported high levels of loneliness. Furthermore, many interventions included loneliness as a secondary outcome and had not been designed explicitly to address loneliness, offering explanations for why 1) the samples did not report loneliness at baseline, and 2) the interventions were not as successful at reducing loneliness as one might hope. Currently, evidence-based interventions are needed that are specifically aimed at young people who report loneliness.

Efforts to target youth with elevated levels of loneliness are hampered by the lack of consensus on cutoff criteria for loneliness measures to distinguish lonely from non-lonely individuals; normed data are also not available, making it difficult to target lonely individuals for intervention. We discussed this issue earlier in this chapter, but now we call for further work on the measurement of youth loneliness with the aim of establishing screening criteria and creating normed data, which is crucial to help inform future interventions.

Case Vignette

Eleanor was a 15-year-old woman with psychiatric history of anorexia nervosa, binge-eating/purging subtype, and no pertinent past medical history who presented for initial evaluation at the child and adolescent psychiatry clinic after completing 12 weeks of residential eating disorder treatment. She was interviewed in conjunction with her mother. Eleanor's mother reported her daughter was a healthy, happy baby who "couldn't get enough time with her mama." Eleanor struggled with attending preschool and kindergarten, often crying and complaining of feeling sick every Monday morning. Her mother reported that this behavior stopped once Eleanor met her first-grade teacher, a thoughtful woman who helped Eleanor adjust to being in school.

Eleanor loved her art and reading classes throughout elementary and junior high school. Eleanor was "always a shy girl" but usually had one or two close friends every year, in addition to being very close with her older brother and loving the family's three pet dogs. Eleanor began struggling when she transitioned to her freshman year on a new high school campus. She began to receive a lot of attention, some negative and some positive, from peers in her class. Her mother noted that the family are "early bloomers" and that Eleanor had been picked on by girls in her new school and made uncomfortable by older boys due to this fact. Eleanor reported this change and feeling out of control as the reasoning for wanting to lose weight, to "just get the comments to stop happening."

Eleanor began restricting intake, counting calories, and going on 1- to 2-hour walks every day. Although she "lost a few pounds," the bullying continued, and she continued to have a hard time making friends at her new school. "At some point," she stated, "I knew losing more weight wasn't really going to make them stop, but by then it felt safer and like the only thing I could control, so I didn't want to stop." Eleanor began forcing herself to vomit in the winter. "I felt so lonely, and like I never was going to have any friends again." Eleanor reported behaviors like this kept happening until the spring and that her mom and brother started noticing as the weather got warmer and "I couldn't hide under big sweaters and coats anymore."

Eleanor was treated in a three-phase recovery and relapse-prevention residential eating disorder center over 3 months in the summer. During the residential treatment, Eleanor was weight-restored rapidly, and much of her treatment focused on family therapy, individual psychotherapy, and initiating medication to help manage her mood and anxiety symptoms. Eleanor followed a step-down model of increasing autonomy regarding eating and exercise behaviors and had not struggled with any restricting, overexercising, or purging for 2 months. She had been back in school for 1 month and was a freshman at a new high school.

When asked about what was the most helpful from her 3-month residential stay, Eleanor stated that beyond learning how to nourish and care for her body, her therapist was really helpful. Eleanor stated that in therapy, "We worked a lot on how I thought my body was bad, and how if I lost weight then I would feel better, and people would be nicer to me." Eleanor's mother agreed that Eleanor had been a lot happier for the past 2 months since treatment began to have a real impact.

When asked about the past month outside of her residential, structured treatment, Eleanor stated that eating how she used to and only exercising in gym class had been pretty easy and that she had not felt a lot of distress about her body lately. When asked about how the new school has been, she reported that this transition "had been a lot less easy." When prompted further, Eleanor stated, "I know I should feel better about this, and my therapist told me I need to be nicer to both my body and myself, but I just feel like I'm never going to make friends. Everyone was so mean to me last year, and I feel like everyone is going to treat me the same way again, especially now that I have this eating disorder diagnosis, I'm even more different. I feel like no one can get me besides the other girls who have been through what I've been through, like the ones in the center were. I've always been shy, but I'm starting to think I just don't know how to make friends, and that I'll always be lonely."

After meeting with Eleanor and her mother and discussing her history, the psychiatrist brought up a few ideas to further help and support Eleanor as she continued to transition from recovery and into the new school. Beyond continuing the antidepressant Eleanor was placed on for anxiety and mood management, a more holistic plan was formulated for the coming months. First, she would continue having weekly, hour-long therapy with her new therapist in the community, who specialized in dialectical behavior therapy (DBT) and worked with adolescents with eating disorders and anxiety disorders. With her weekly therapy, Eleanor could keep working on challenging her thoughts that things would "always be" one way or the other, including her feelings of loneliness. Eleanor and her therapist would also work on a stepwise approach to challenging her social anxieties, first in small, safe ways at school and then in larger ways by reaching out to new classmates and friends for one-on-one plans to increase her supports and challenge the negative cognition that she would always be bullied. She would also learn more DBT skills for when she was very upset and feeling "the most lonely." Together, challenging Eleanor's defeating cognitions and creating more skills to handle feeling isolated would continue to support her recovery.

Secondly, Eleanor and her mother were given contacts for an adolescent-centered body image and eating disorder recovery group online that met once every 2 weeks via Zoom and was led by a therapist. Eleanor would be able to engage with a community that understands the struggle of recovering from an eating disorder. In this sphere, Eleanor would be able to feel connected and less isolated with her diagnosis and struggles and be able to connect with others who understand while being supported in a safe environment by a guiding group leader.

Lastly, at the community level, Eleanor mentioned the arts and activities she enjoyed previously at school and while in treatment. Although it may be overwhelming initially, one of the goals for her with her therapist, family, and psychiatrist would be to try taking a pottery class next fall after school, where she could deepen her natural talent and connect with others who enjoy the same things she does. This would also act as another community for Eleanor to be known and seen in and to connect with others over what she finds meaningful.

In children and adolescents, chronic illness, poor mental health, and eating disorders can be bidirectionally related to feelings of loneliness. Treatment and management of the primary illness, as well as specific support and communities of understanding, can be of help in combating the sense of isolation from peers. Psychotherapeutically, teaching patients how to question thought distortions that are self-defeating and lead to a negative spiral toward isolation (i.e., all or nothing, personalization of social mistreatment) can benefit patients and increase a sense of empowerment and self-esteem. These cognitive skills can help patients discard maladaptive social cognitions about self and belonging and thus can decrease the barrier to forming new relationships and maintaining ongoing ones. Involvement in community groups that involve skill building and practicing social challenge can improve mastery, build connections, and be an easier source of entry for friendship than some high school settings.

Summary

In this chapter, we highlighted the fact that risk factors for youth loneliness have been addressed through interventions and evaluated systematically using pre/post and RCT designs. The evaluated interventions focus primarily on individual difference, interpersonal, and situational risk factors targeting social and emotional skills development, social isolation, and social support. Of course, those foci could reduce loneliness by improving the quality of relationships and increasing companionship, meaningful connections, belongingness, and empathic understanding, but the success of such interventions is varied.

One consistent finding is the success of psychological therapy as an intervention for youth loneliness. The focus of such interventions is on the management of the maladaptive cognitions associated with loneliness and the adoption of adaptive coping strategies. Although this is key when loneliness stems from such deficits, our review highlights other factors that need to be addressed. In particular is the absence of interventions addressing the sociocultural factors linked to youth loneliness. Attention to such risk factors requires an interdisciplinary commitment to improve transportation links, improve housing, provide welcoming (and well-maintained) meeting spaces in residential areas, restore community cohesion, and promote inclusive environments. Thus, tackling loneliness goes beyond individuals and their immediate relationships; interventions must recognize and address other aspects of the system or systems in which social relationships take place. These more complex interventions will require thought, but they have the potential to increase the number and strength of social networks within communities, and those connections can serve as both personal and community resources for reducing loneliness.

KEY POINTS

- Loneliness among children and adolescents is associated prospectively with depression, social anxiety, and self-harm and has been linked detrimentally with self-reported health and sleep and with low academic performance and job struggles.

- Risk factors span the individual, interpersonal, situational, and sociocultural levels.

- To date, only a handful of interventions focused on youth loneliness have been successful at reducing loneliness.

- Of the tested interventions, psychological therapy appears to be the most useful for youth.

- There is a need for the systematic evaluation of interventions that focus on sociocultural risk factors and more robust evaluation of interventions for youth reporting loneliness.

Suggested Readings

Barreto M, Victor C, Hammond C, et al: Loneliness around the world: age, gender, and cultural differences in loneliness. Pers Individ Dif 169:110066, 2021 33536694

Eccles AM, Qualter P: Review: Alleviating loneliness in young people: a meta-analysis of interventions. Child Adolesc Ment Health 26(1):17–33, 2021 32406165

Qualter P, Vanhalst J, Harris R, et al: Loneliness across the life span. Perspect Psychol Sci 10(2):250–264, 2015 25910393

Watson R, Sellars E, Qualter P, et al: Brief: evidence-informed recommendations for supporting young people with feeling lonely, isolated, and disconnected. CoRAY, January 1, 2021. Available at: https://emergingminds.org.uk/wp-content/uploads/2021/01/Co-RAY-Briefing-Loneliness-Isolation-Version-1.0.pdf. Accessed February 2022.

References

Adams KB, Sanders S, Auth EA: Loneliness and depression in independent living retirement communities: risk and resilience factors. Aging Ment Health 8(6):475–485, 2004 15724829

Agadullina ER, Lovakov A, Kiselnikova NV: Does quitting social networks change feelings of loneliness among freshmen? An experimental study. Journal of Applied Research in Higher Education 13(1):149–163, 2020

Alasmawi K, Mann F, Lewis G, et al: To what extent does severity of loneliness vary among different mental health diagnostic groups: a cross-sectional study. Int J Ment Health Nurs 29(5):921–934, 2020 32356331

Anderson CA: Attributional style, depression, and loneliness: a cross-cultural comparison of American and Chinese students. Pers Soc Psychol Bull 25(4):482–499, 1999

Asher SR, Hymel S, Renshaw PD: Loneliness in children. Child Dev 55(4):1456–1464, 1984

Bangee M, Harris RA, Bridges N, et al: Loneliness and attention to social threat in adults: findings from an eye-tracker study. Pers Individ Dif 63:16–23, 2014

Barreto M, Doyle DM, Bhattacharjee P, et al: The impact of everyday stigma on loneliness across identities and countries. Unpublished manuscript, 2021a

Barreto M, Van Breen J, Victor C, et al: Exploring the nature and variation of the stigma associated with loneliness. Unpublished manuscript, 2021b

Barreto M, Victor C, Hammond C, et al: Loneliness around the world: age, gender, and cultural differences in loneliness. Pers Individ Dif 169:110066, 2021c 33536694

Barry TD, Klinger LG, Lee JM, et al: Examining the effectiveness of an outpatient clinic-based social skills group for high-functioning children with autism. J Autism Dev Disord 33(6):685–701, 2003 14714936

Battles HB, Wiener LS: STARBRIGHT World: effects of an electronic network on the social environment of children with life-threatening illnesses. Child Health Care 31(1):47–68, 2002

Beidel DC, Turner SM, Morris TL: Behavioral treatment of childhood social phobia. J Consult Clin Psychol 68(6):1072–1080, 2000 11142541

Borys S, Perlman D: Gender differences in loneliness. Pers Soc Psychol Bull 11:63–74, 1985

Bostick D, Anderson R: Evaluating a small-group counseling program: a model for program planning and improvement in the elementary setting. Professional School Counseling 12(6):428–433, 2009

Bradley R: "Why single me out?" Peer mentoring, autism and inclusion in mainstream secondary schools. British Journal of Special Education 43(3):272–288, 2016

Brouzos A, Vassilopoulos SP, Moschou K: Utilizing storytelling to promote emotional well-being of children with a distinct physical appearance: the case of children who wear eyeglasses. European Journal of Counselling Psychology 4:62–76, 2016

Bueckner S, Maes M, Denissen JJA, Luhmann M: Loneliness and the big five personality traits: a meta-analysis. Eur J Pers 34:8–28, 2020

Chipuer HM, Pretty GH: Facets of adolescents' loneliness: a study of rural and urban Australian youth. Aust Psychol 35(3):233–237, 2000

Christian BJ, D'Auria JP: Building life skills for children with cystic fibrosis: effectiveness of an intervention. Nurs Res 55(5):300–307, 2006 16980830

Christiansen J, Qualter P, Pedersen SS, et al: Associations of loneliness and social isolation with physical and mental health among adolescents and young adults. Perspect Public Health 141(4):226–236, 2021 34148462

Cole A, Bond C, Qualter P, Maes M: A systematic review of the development and psychometric properties of loneliness measures for children and adolescents. Int J Environ Res Public Health 18(6):3285, 2021 33810076

Craig AB, Brown ER, Upright J, DeRosier MF: Enhancing children's social emotional functioning through virtual game-based delivery of social skill training. J Child Fam Stud 25:959–968, 2016

Cross D, Shaw T, Epstein M, et al: Impact of the Friendly Schools whole-school intervention on transition to secondary school and adolescent bullying behaviour. Eur J Educ 53:495–513, 2018

Davis SK, Nowland R, Qualter P: The role of emotional intelligence in the maintenance of depression symptoms and loneliness among children. Front Psychol 10:1672, 2019 31379688

Deckers A, Muris P, Roelofs J, Arntz A: A group-administered social skills training for 8- to 12- year-old, high-functioning children with autism spectrum disorders: an evaluation of its effectiveness in a naturalistic outpatient treatment setting. J Autism Dev Disord 46(11):3493–3504, 2016 27522220

Deri S, Davidai S, Gilovich T: Home alone: why people believe others' social lives are richer than their own. J Pers Soc Psychol 113(6):858–877, 2017 29189037

Diab M, Punamäki R-L, Palosaari E, Qouta SR: Can psychosocial intervention improve peer and sibling relations among war-affected children? Impact and mediating analyses in a randomized controlled trial. Soc Dev 23(2):215–231, 2014

Doyle DM, Barreto M: Social stigma increases loneliness among ethnic minorities. Unpublished manuscript, 2021

Doyle DM, Molix L: Disparities in social health by sexual orientation and the etiologic role of self-reported discrimination. Arch Sex Behav 45(6):1317–1327, 2016 26566900

Eccles AM, Qualter P: Review: alleviating loneliness in young people: a meta-analysis of interventions. Child Adolesc Ment Health 26(1):17–33, 2021 32406165

Eccles AM, Qualter P, Madsen KR, Holstein BE: Loneliness in the lives of Danish adolescents: associations with health and sleep. Scand J Public Health 48(8):877–887, 2020 31969070

Frankel F, Myatt R, Sugar C, et al: A randomized controlled study of parent-assisted Children's Friendship Training with children having autism spectrum disorders. J Autism Dev Disord 40(7):827–842, 2010 20058059

Gantman A, Kapp SK, Orenski K, Laugeson EA: Social skills training for young adults with high-functioning autism spectrum disorders: a randomized controlled pilot study. J Autism Dev Disord 42(6):1094–1103, 2012 21915740

Grace E, Raghavendra P, Newman L, et al: Learning to use the internet and online social media: what is the effectiveness of home-based intervention for youth with complex communication needs? Child Lang Teach Ther 30(2):141–157, 2014

Halpin SA, Allen MW: Changes in psychosocial well-being during stages of gay identity development. J Homosex 47(2):109–126, 2004 15271626

Harris RA, Qualter P, Robinson SJ: Loneliness trajectories from middle childhood to pre-adolescence: impact on perceived health and sleep disturbance. J Adolesc 36(6):1295–1304, 2013 23403089

Heu LC, van Zomeren M, Hansen N: Lonely alone or lonely together? A cultural-psychological examination of individualism-collectivism and loneliness in five European countries. Pers Soc Psychol Bull 45(5):780–793, 2019 30264659

Hunt MG, Marx R, Lipson C, Young J: No more FOMO: limiting social media decreases loneliness and depression. J Soc Clin Psychol 37(10):751–768, 2018

Iffland B, Sansen LM, Catani C, Neuner F: The trauma of peer abuse: effects of relational peer victimization and social anxiety disorder on physiological and affective reactions to social exclusion. Front Psychiatry 5:26, 2014 24672491

Jackson T: Protective self-presentation, sources of socialization, and loneliness among Australian adolescents and young adults. Pers Individ Dif 43:1552–1562, 2007

Jeon YH, Kraus SG, Jowsey T, et al: The experience of living with chronic heart failure: a narrative review of qualitative studies. BMC Health Serv Res 10:77, 2010

Jobe-Shields L, Cohen R, Parra GR: Patterns of change in children's loneliness: trajectories from third through fifth grades. Merril-Palmer Quarterly 57(1):25–47, 2011

Jones WH, Freemon JE, Goswick RA: The persistence of loneliness: self and other determinants. J Pers 49:27–48, 1981

Kearns A, Whitley E, Tannahill C, Ellaway A: Loneliness, social relations and health and well-being in deprived communities. Psychol Health Med 20(3):332–344, 2015 25058303

Kidd SA: Youth homelessness and social stigma. J Youth Adolesc 36(3):291–299, 2007 27519028

Kim SY, Bottema-Beutel K: Negotiation of individual and collective identities in the online discourse of autistic adults. Autism in Adulthood 1(1):69–78, 2019

King GA, Specht JA, Schultz I, et al: Social skills training for withdrawn unpopular children with physical disabilities: a preliminary evaluation. Rehabil Psychol 42(1):47–60, 1997

Kjøbli J, Ogden T: A randomized effectiveness trial of individual child social skills training: six-month follow-up. Child Adolesc Psychiatry Ment Health 8(1):31, 2014 25614762

Klimstra TA, Luyckx K, Branje S, et al: Personality traits, interpersonal identity, and relationship stability: longitudinal linkages in late adolescence and young adulthood. J Youth Adolesc 42(11):1661–1673, 2013 23149696

Klingman A, Hochdorf Z: Coping with distress and self harm: the impact of a primary prevention program among adolescents. J Adolesc 16(2):121–140, 1993 8376638

Kneer J, van Eldik AK, Jansz J, et al: With a little help from my friends: peer coaching for refugee adolescents and the role of social media. Media Commun 7(2):264–274, 2019

Kochenderfer-Ladd B, Wardrop JL: Chronicity and instability of children's peer victimization experiences as predictors of loneliness and social satisfaction trajectories. Child Dev 72(1):134–151, 2001 11280475

Kopelman-Rubin D, Klomek AB, Al-Yagon M, et al: Psychological intervention for adolescents diagnosed with learning disorders—"I Can Succeed" (ICS): treatment model, feasibility, and acceptability. Int J Res Learn Disabil 1(1):37–54, 2012

Krabbe J, Forkmann T: Frequency vs. intensity: which should be used as anchors for self-report instruments? Health Qual Life Outcomes 10:107, 2012

Ladd GW, Ettekal I: Peer-related loneliness across early to late adolescence: normative trends, intra-individual trajectories, and links with depressive symptoms. J Adolesc 36(6):1269–1282, 2013 23787076

Larsen TB, Urke H, Tobro M, et al: Promoting mental health and preventing loneliness in upper secondary school in Norway: effects of a randomized controlled trial. Scandinavian Journal of Educational Research 65(2):181–194, 2019

Lasgaard M, Nielsen A, Eriksen ME, Goossens L: Loneliness and social support in adolescent boys with autism spectrum disorders. J Autism Dev Disord 40(2):218–226, 2010 19685285

Lasgaard M, Goossens L, Elklit A: Loneliness, depressive symptomatology, and suicide ideation in adolescence: cross-sectional and longitudinal analyses. J Abnorm Child Psychol 39(1):137–150, 2011 20700646

Lasgaard M, Friis K, Shevlin M: "Where are all the lonely people?" A population-based study of high-risk groups across the life span. Soc Psychiatry Psychiatr Epidemiol 51(10):1373–1384, 2016 27571769

Laursen B, Hartl AC: Understanding loneliness during adolescence: developmental changes that increase the risk of perceived social isolation. J Adolesc 36(6):1261–1268, 2013 23866959

Lee SY: How do people compare themselves with others on social network sites? The case of Facebook. Comput Human Behav 32:253–260, 2014

Leff SS, Gullan RL, Paskewich BS, et al: An initial evaluation of a culturally adapted social problem-solving and relational aggression prevention program for urban African-American relationally aggressive girls. J Prev Interv Community 37(4):260–274, 2009 19830622

Lev-Wiesel R, Sternberg R: Victimized at home re-victimized by peers: domestic child abuse a risk factor for social rejection. Child Adolesc Social Work J 29(3):203–220, 2012

Leventhal T, Brooks-Gunn J: The neighborhoods they live in: the effects of neighborhood residence on child and adolescent outcomes. Psychol Bull 126(2):309–337, 2000 10748645

Levine MP: Loneliness and eating disorders. J Psychol 146(1–2):243–257, 2012 22303623

Levitt HM, Ippolito MR: Being transgender: the experience of transgender identity development. J Homosex 61(12):1727–1758, 2014 25089681

Lim MH, Rodebaugh TL, Eres R, et al: A pilot digital intervention targeting loneliness in youth mental health. Front Psychiatry 10:604, 2019 31507469

Loades ME, Chatburn E, Higson-Sweeney N, et al: Rapid systematic review: the impact of social isolation and loneliness on the mental health of children and adolescents in the context of COVID-19. J Am Acad Child Adolesc Psychiatry 59(11):1218–1239, 2020 32504808

Long CR, Averill JR: Solitude: an exploration of benefits of being alone. J Theory Soc Behav 33(1):21–44, 2003

Luhmann M, Hawkley LC: Age differences in loneliness from late adolescence to oldest old age. Dev Psychol 52(6):943–959, 2016 27148782

Lykes VA, Kemmelmeier M: What predicts loneliness? Cultural difference between individualistic and collectivist societies in Europe. J Cross Cult Psychol 45(2):468–490, 2014

Madsen KR, Damsgaard MT, Rubin M, et al: Loneliness and ethnic composition of the school class: a nationally random sample of adolescents. J Youth Adolesc 45(7):1350–1365, 2016 26861709

Madsen KR, Holstein BE, Damsgaard MT, et al: Trends in social inequality in loneliness among adolescents 1991–2014. J Public Health (Oxf) 41(2):e133–e140, 2019 30053062

Maes M, Vanhalst J, Spithoven AWM, et al: Loneliness and attitudes toward aloneness in adolescence: a person-centered approach. J Youth Adolesc 45(3):547–567, 2016 26369350

Maes M, Van den Noortgate W, Fustolo-Gunnink SF, et al: Loneliness in children and adolescents with chronic physical conditions: a meta-analysis. J Pediatr Psychol 42(6):622–635, 2017 28340072

Maes M, Qualter P, Vanhalst J, et al: Gender differences in loneliness across the lifespan: a meta-analysis. Eur J Pers 33:642–654, 2019

Marcoen A, Goossens L, Caes P: Lonelines in pre- through late adolescence: exploring the contributions of a multidimensional approach. J Youth Adolesc 16(6):561–577, 1987 24277491

Margalit M: Effects of social skills training for students with an intellectual disability. International Journal of Disability, Development and Education 42(1):75–85, 1995a

Margalit M: Social skills learning for students with learning disabilities and students with behaviour disorders. Educ Psychol 15(4):445–456, 1995b

Masi CM, Chen HY, Hawkley LC, Cacioppo JT: A meta-analysis of interventions to reduce loneliness. Pers Soc Psychol Rev 15(3):219–266, 2011 20716644

Masia-Warner C, Klein RG, Dent HC, et al: School-based intervention for adolescents with social anxiety disorder: results of a controlled study. J Abnorm Child Psychol 33(6):707–722, 2005 16328746

Mason M, Zaharakis N, Sabo R: Reducing social stress in urban adolescents with peer network counseling. J Child Fam Stud 25(12):3488–3496, 2016

Mattanah JF, Ayers JF, Brand BL, et al: A social support intervention to ease the college transition: exploring main effects and moderators. Journal of College Student Development 51(1):93–108, 2010

Matthews NL, Orr BC, Warriner K, et al: Exploring the effectiveness of a peer-mediated model of the peers curriculum: a pilot randomized control trial. J Autism Dev Disord 48(7):2458–2475, 2018 29453708

Matthews T, Danese A, Gregory AM, et al: Sleeping with one eye open: loneliness and sleep quality in young adults. Psychol Med 47(12):2177–2186, 2017 28511734

Matthews T, Danese A, Caspi A, et al: Lonely young adults in modern Britain: findings from an epidemiological cohort study. Psychol Med 49(2):268–277, 2019a 29684289

Matthews T, Odgers CL, Danese A, et al: Loneliness and neighborbood characteristics: a multi-informant, nationally representative study of young adults. Psychol Sci 30(5):765–775, 2019b 30955415

Matthews T, Caspi A, Danese A, et al: A longitudinal twin study of victimization and loneliness from childhood to young adulthood. Dev Psychopathol 34(1):367–377, 2022 33046153

Mazumdar S, Learnihan V, Cochrane T, Davey R: The built environment and social capital: a systematic review. Environ Behav 50(2):119–158, 2018

Merz EM, Jak S: The long reach of childhood: childhood experiences influence close relationships and loneliness across life. Adv Life Course Res 18(3):212–222, 2013 24796560

Nightingale SM, Roberts S, Tariq V, et al: Trajectories of university adjustment in the United Kingdom: emotion management and emotional self-efficacy protect against initial poor adjustment. Learn Individ Differ 27:174–181, 2013

Nowland R, Necka EA, Cacioppo JT: Loneliness and social internet use: pathways to reconnection in a digital world? Perspect Psychol Sci 13(1):70–87, 2018 28937910

Office for National Statistics: Loneliness: what characteristics and circumstances are associated with feeling lonely? London, Office for National Statistics, 2018. Available at: www.ons.gov.uk/peoplepopulationandcommunity/wellbeing/articles/lonelinesswhatcharacteristicsandcircumstancesareassociatedwithfeelinglonely/2018-04-10. Accessed July 27, 2019.

Pempek TA, Yermolayeva YA, Calvert SL: College students' social networking experiences on Facebook. J Appl Dev Psychol 30(3):227–238, 2009

Petrina N, Carter M, Stephenson J, Sweller N: Friendship satisfaction in children with autism spectrum disorder and nominated friends. J Autism Dev Disord 47(2):384–392, 2017 27866352

Priest N, Perry R, Ferdinand A, et al: Effects over time of self-reported direct and vicarious racial discrimination on depressive symptoms and loneliness among Australian school students. BMC Psychiatry 17(1):50, 2017 28159001

Purohit SP, Pradhan B, Nagendra HR: Effect of yoga on EUROFIT physical fitness parameters on adolescents dwelling in an orphan home: a randomized control study. Vulnerable Child Youth Stud 11(1):33–46, 2016

Qualter P, Munn P: The separateness of social and emotional loneliness in childhood. J Child Psychol Psychiatry 43:233–244, 2002 11902602

Qualter P, Brown SL, Rotenberg KJ, et al: Trajectories of loneliness during childhood and adolescence: predictors and health outcomes. J Adolesc 36(6):1283–1293, 2013a 23465384

Qualter P, Rotenberg K, Barrett L, et al: Investigating hypervigilance for social threat of lonely children. J Abnorm Child Psychol 41(2):325–338, 2013b 22956297

Qualter P, Vanhalst J, Harris R, et al: Loneliness across the life span. Perspect Psychol Sci 10(2):250–264, 2015 25910393

Qualter P, Hennessey A, Yang K, et al: Trends in the experience of loneliness among U.K. adolescents 2002–2014: associations with social inequality, health, and educational outcomes. Unpublished manuscript, 2021a

Qualter P, Victor C, Hammond C, et al: Predictors of frequency, intensity, and duration of loneliness: latent profile analyses of data from the BBC Loneliness Experiment. Unpublished manuscript, 2021b

Quayle D, Dziurawiec S, Roberts C, et al: The effect of an optimism and lifeskills program on depressive symptoms in preadolescence. Behav Change 18(4):194–203, 2001

Ravenscroft J, Wazny K, Davis JM: Factors associated with successful transition among children with disabilities in eight European countries. PLoS One 12(6):e0179904, 2017 28636649

Regev D, Guttmann J: The psychological benefits of artwork: the case of children with learning disorders. Arts Psychother 32:302–312, 2005

Renshaw PD, Brown PJ: Loneliness in middle childhood: concurrent and longitudinal predictors. Child Dev 64:1271–1284, 1993

Roberts RE, Lewinsohn PM, Seeley JR: A brief measure of loneliness suitable for use with adolescents. Psychol Rep 72(3):1379–1391, 1993

Rohde P, Jorgensen JS, Seeley JR, Mace DE: Pilot evaluation of the Coping Course: a cognitive-behavioral intervention to enhance coping skills in incarcerated youth. J Am Acad Child Adolesc Psychiatry 43(6):669–676, 2004 15167083

Rotenberg KJ, Addis N, Betts LR, et al: The relation between trust beliefs and loneliness during early childhood, middle childhood, and adulthood. Pers Soc Psychol Bull 36(8):1086–1100, 2010 20585058

Russell D, Peplau LA, Ferguson M: Developing measures of loneliness. J Pers 48:290–294, 1978

Sanchez R, Brown E, Kocher K, DeRosier M: Improving children's mental health with a digital social skills development game: a randomized controlled efficacy trial of adventures aboard the S.S. GRIN. Games Health J 6(1):19–27, 2017 28051877

Schinka KC, van Dulmen MHM, Mata AD, et al: Psychosocial predictors and outcomes of loneliness trajectories from childhood to early adolescence. J Adolesc 36(6):1251–1260, 2013 24007942

Shiovitz-Ezra S, Ayalon L: Use of direct versus indirect approaches to measure loneliness in later life. Res Aging 34:572–591, 2012

Smith NG, Hart TA, Kidwai A, et al: Results of a pilot study to ameliorate psychological and behavioral outcomes of minority stress among young gay and bisexual men. Behav Ther 48(5):664–677, 2017 28711116

Sosnowy C, Silverman C, Shattuck P: Parents' and young adults' perspectives on transition outcomes for young adults with autism. Autism 22(1):29–39, 2018

Stewart M, Barnfather A, Magill-Evans J, et al: Brief report: an online support intervention: perceptions of adolescents with physical disabilities. J Adolesc 34(4):795–800, 2011 20488511

Stewart M, Letourneau N, Masuda JR, et al: Impacts of online peer support for children with asthma and allergies: "it just helps you every time you can't breathe well." J Pediatr Nurs 28(5):439–452, 2013 23398896

Stice E, Rohde P, Seeley JR, Gau JM: Testing mediators of intervention effects in randomized controlled trials: an evaluation of three depression prevention programs. J Consult Clin Psychol 78(2):273–280, 2010 20350038

Thomas L, Orme E, Kerrigan F: Student loneliness: the role of social media through life transitions. Comput Educ 146:103754, 2020

Tough H, Siegrist J, Fekete C: Social relationships, mental health and wellbeing in physical disability: a systematic review. BMC Public Health 17(1):414, 2017 28482878

Uskul AK, Over H: Culture, social interdependence, and ostracism. Curr Dir Psychol Sci 26(4):371–376, 2017 van Roekel E, Scholte RHJ, Engels RCME, et al: Loneliness in the daily lives of adolescents: an experience sampling study examining the effects of social contexts. J Early Adolesc 35:905–930, 2015

Vanhalst J, Goossens L, Luyckx K, et al: The development of loneliness from mid- to late adolescence: trajectory classes, personality traits, and psychosocial functioning. J Adolesc 36(6):1305–1312, 2013a 22560517

Vanhalst J, Luyckx K, Scholte RHJ, et al: Low self-esteem as a risk factor for loneliness in adolescence: perceived—but not actual—social acceptance as an underlying mechanism. J Abnorm Child Psychol 41(7):1067–1081, 2013b 23661185

Vanhalst J, Luyckx K, Goossens L: Experiencing loneliness in adolescence: a matter of individual characteristics, negative peer experiences, or both? Soc Dev 23:100–118, 2014

Vanhalst J, Soenens B, Luyckx K, et al: Why do the lonely stay lonely? Chronically lonely adolescents' attributions and emotions in situations of social inclusion and exclusion. J Pers Soc Psychol 109(5):932–948, 2015 26191959

Vassilopoulos S, Diakogiorgi K, Brouzos A, et al: A problem-oriented group approach to reduce children's fears and concerns about the secondary school transition. J Psychol Couns Sch 28(1):84–101, 2018

Victor C, Grenade L, Boldy D: Loneliness in later life: a comparison of differing measures. Rev Clin Gerontol 15:63–70, 2005

Vogel EA, Rose JP, Okdie BM, et al: Who compares and despairs? The effect of social comparison orientation on social media use and its outcomes. Pers Individ Dif 86:249–256, 2015

Wang JM, Rubin KH, Laursen B, et al: Preference-for-solitude and adjustment difficulties in early and late adolescence. J Clin Child Adolesc Psychol 42(6):834–842, 2013 23682608

Wang J, Lloyd-Evans B, Marston L, et al: Loneliness as a predictor of outcomes in mental disorders among people who have experienced a mental health crisis: a 4-month prospective study. BMC Psychiatry 20(1):249, 2020 32434492

Yang K, Petersen KJ, Qualter P: Undesirable social relations as risk factors for loneliness among 14-year-olds in the UK: findings from the Millennium Cohort Study. Int J Behav Dev 46(1):3–9, 2022

Zhang N, Fan F, Huang S, Rodriquez MA: Mindfulness training for loneliness among Chinese college students: a pilot randomized controlled trial. Int J Psychol 53(5):373–378, 2016 27704544

Zhao S, Grasmuck S, Martin J: Identity construction on Facebook: digital empowerment in anchored relationships. Comput Human Behav 24(5):1816–1836, 2008

Zimmer-Gembeck MJ, Trevaskis S, Nesdale D, Downey GA: Relational victimization, loneliness and depressive symptoms: indirect associations via self and peer reports of rejection sensitivity. J Youth Adolesc 43(4):568–582, 2014 23955324

9

Interventions for Loneliness in Older Adults

Kimberly A. Van Orden, Ph.D.
Yeates Conwell, M.D.

PEOPLE AROUND THE WORLD are living longer, and the number of older adults in the United States and worldwide is on the rise— a phenomenon known as "population aging" (Kinsella and Wan 2009; United Nations 2009). Globally, in 2018 the number of older adults (age 65 and older) was greater than the number of children age 5 or younger for the first time in history, and projections indicate that by 2050, there will be more older adults than younger people ages 15–24 (U.N. Department of Economic and Social Affairs). Addressing health and well-being for older adults must be a significant priority in health care and for policy makers given these changes in demography. *Social health*—the degree to which an older person can meaningfully participate in activities, fulfill social roles, and engage with others (Huber et al. 2011)—may be an especially import-ant domain of health and a target for interventions in later life to promote quality of life, given that social health remains malleable throughout life even in the context of physical, cognitive, and sensory limitations. Indeed, older adults place a greater priority on social relationships than younger adults and tend to report greater relationship satisfaction, more frequent positive emotions, and greater skill with managing emotions than younger adults (Carstensen et al. 2011; Charles and Carstensen 2010; Scheibe and Carstensen 2010). Social health is an aging-related strength that can be capitalized upon to compensate for declines in other areas of health and functioning. Social connection matters in later life to ensure that quality of life is maintained and thus is a key public health target (Holt-Lunstad 2021; Holt-Lunstad et al. 2017). Social connections that create a sense of caring, contributing, and community have a range of benefits for health and well-being and can protect against loneliness and declines in mental health and quality of life (Blazer 2020).

Although the size of social networks reliably declines with age, much of this change is due to an active process of "pruning" one's networks to prioritize the most meaningful relationships (Charles and Carstensen 2010). A loss of relationships through death becomes increasingly important with advancing age, but although the number of people in older adults' networks is smaller than at earlier developmental stages, loneliness and social isolation are not normative experiences in later life. Still, a significant portion of older adults do not follow the trajectory of healthy aging and do experience loneliness, with estimates ranging from 11% to 43%, with greater prevalence in mental health and long-term care settings (Anderson 2010; Heikkinen and Kauppinen 2011; Holmén and Furukawa 2002; Jylhä 2004; Perissinotto et al. 2012; Rubenowitz et al. 2001; Steptoe et al. 2013; Victor and Bowling 2012; Wenger and Burholt 2004). Research with older adults has confirmed that loneliness is due in part to objective circumstances—increasing disability and frailty, environmental barriers to socialization, and bereavement—and to subjective perceptions (e.g., low self-esteem, social anxiety) and ineffective emotion regulation strategies that cause and perpetuate loneliness (Aartsen and Jylhä 2011; Cacioppo et al. 2014; Cohen-Mansfield et al. 2016; Hoogendijk et al. 2016; Preece et al. 2021; Qualter et al. 2015; Theeke 2010).

Loneliness in older adults is both an indicator (or component) of and a determinant of (or contributor to) deficits in healthy aging. Theory and empirical data indicate that humans have an innate "need to belong" to social relationships and groups. When this need is not met, loneliness emerges. Loneliness is distressing and an indicator that an older adult is not on a healthy aging trajectory, that the person perceives their social world as lacking and deficient and the person's need to belong is not being met.

There are three forms of loneliness, each of which points to a different component of an older adult's social world that is insufficient (Cacioppo et al. 2015; Weiss 1973). *Emotional* (or intimate) loneliness indicates the lack of a significant person (e.g., spouse, best friend, close confidant) on whom the older adult can rely for emotional support during times of stress. For older adults, losing a spouse is associated with intimate loneliness (Cacioppo et al. 2015). *Social* (or relational) loneliness is caused by a perceived absence of close ties to friends and family. For older adults, low social engagement— a lack of frequent and satisfying social contacts—is associated with relational loneliness. *Collective* loneliness refers to an absence of perceived connectedness with a larger, meaningful group (e.g., volunteer group, church choir, golf league). For older adults, a low amount of (or absence of) participation in voluntary organizations is associated with collective loneliness (Cacioppo et al. 2015).

As a determinant, the effects of loneliness on well-being, health, and premature mortality are robust, supported by numerous longitudinal studies conducted over several decades by diverse research groups (Cacioppo and Hawkley 2003; Tomaka et al. 2006). Specifically, loneliness in later life is associated with reduced quality of life, including well-being and depressive symptoms (Cacioppo et al. 2010; Golden et al. 2009); unhealthy behaviors, such as smoking, an unhealthy diet, and a lack of exercise (Hawkley et al. 2009; Shankar et al. 2011; Whisman 2010); and adverse health outcomes, including cardiovascular disease, metabolic syndrome, hypertension, pain, fatigue, insomnia, depression, dementia, suicide, and all-cause mortality (Cacioppo et al. 2010; Hawkley et al. 2010; Holwerda et al. 2014; Luo et al. 2012; Steptoe et al. 2013; Waern et al. 2003; Whisman 2010). The risk of premature mortality due to loneliness is comparable to the risk of maintaining an unhealthy diet, physical inactivity, alcohol misuse, and smoking and is associated with increased health care utilization (Gerst-Emerson and Jayawardhana 2015). However, loneliness in older age may be more amenable to cost-effective intervention than other health behaviors, spurring its emergence as a bona fide public health problem and a focus for development of preventive interventions (Gerst-Emerson and Jayawardhana 2015; Holt-Lunstad et al. 2010).

Scant data are available indicating that any intervention (behavioral or pharmacological) is reliably effective in reducing loneliness. Few intervention studies have examined this outcome, and those that have been conducted commonly have design flaws (Cohen and Janicki-Deverts 2009; Findlay 2003). Nonetheless, systematic and meta-analytic reviews suggest that it is possible for behavioral interventions to reduce loneliness in later life. A meta-analysis of 50 clinical trials of behavioral interventions to decrease loneliness in adults found that those interventions that employed psychotherapy to specifically address loneliness using social cognitive strategies were the most effective, although the effect was small (Masi et al. 2011). This meta-analysis, although important, has limitations regarding its generalization to older adults experiencing loneliness. First, samples included adults of all ages. Second, subjects did not have to report clinically significant loneliness at study entry. Third, most studies were not randomized. Fourth, many studies utilized psychotherapy, which may be a less useful approach for older adults because they are less likely to receive mental health care outside of primary care settings.

Systematic reviews of interventions to reduce loneliness in older adults suggest that group educational/support interventions and use of technology may be effective, but all reviews highlight the need for further research with rigorous experimental designs and delineation of key elements and mechanisms of action (Cattan et al. 2005; Cohen-Mansfield and Perach 2015; Dickens et al. 2011; Findlay 2003; Hagan et al. 2014; O'Rourke et al. 2018). Some approaches appear promising to prevent or reduce loneliness in older adults, but there is not enough empirical evidence to date to clearly identify any given program as evidence-based to reduce or prevent loneliness in later life, for the following reasons: First, no studies have replicated findings for efficacious programs. Second, most programs tested did not provide standardized programs, thus limiting effective dissemination and implementation with fidelity. Third, most studies to date have not enrolled lonely older adults, which may limit findings because individuals experiencing loneliness may find programs more or less acceptable than those who are not lonely (Stuart et al. 2022). Fourth, community providers suggest that more research attention should be paid to understanding the relevance of programs to a given older adult and the acceptability of programs to address loneliness, with the goal of improving their uptake and utilization (Sabir et al. 2009).

One means by which to address these limitations is by organizing available programs by the pathway to loneliness that they may most effectively target. Loneliness results from several interconnected pathways in later life, including poor mental health, poor physical health, reduced cognitive functioning, reduced physical functioning, and social stressors. We hypothesize that the acceptability and effectiveness of programs for older adults will be impacted by individualized pathways to loneliness. Thus, tailoring the selection of programs to individual preferences and clinical need may increase benefit.

Interventions for Loneliness in Later Life

A one-size-fits-all approach to promoting social connections is unlikely to be effective or acceptable to lonely older adults, but the evidence base to support one intervention over another is limited (Holt-Lunstad et al. 2017). Considering personalized contributing factors to loneliness as well as factors that impact ability and willingness to engage in an intervention may re-

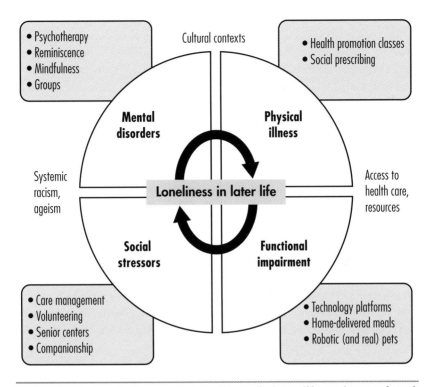

FIGURE 9–1. Pathways to loneliness in later life and associated interventions.

sult in better outcomes. In this chapter, we discuss the current evidence base for programs to prevent or reduce loneliness in later life using a conceptualization of available programs based on their suitability or relevance to a given pathway to loneliness. This conceptualization is intended to generate ideas and directions for future research and to assist clinicians in selecting programs for clinical need in the absence of a clear evidence base. The model (Figure 9–1) includes four broad domains that represent key contributors (or pathways) to loneliness in later life, as well as corresponding intervention approaches that may be useful to address loneliness in those circumstances. Interventions we selected have at least some empirical evidence to support them as promising or effective.

One pathway to loneliness is via *mental health* symptoms or disorders. Older adults who experience depression, anxiety, and other mental health disorders are at greater risk for loneliness. Another pathway is via *physical health* symptoms or illnesses; older adults who report poor self-perceived health and a greater number of chronic conditions are at increased risk for loneliness. Impairments in physical, cognitive, and sensory *function* are also associated with increased risk for loneliness in later life, including reduced mobility, impairments in self-care, reduced physical strength, declines in memory, impairments in executive functioning, and loss of vision and hearing. A lack of social resources and the presence of *social stressors* are also associated with loneliness in later life, including bereavement, lack of transportation, financial insecurity, relocation to senior living facilities, retirement, and low social support. These domains of risk interact and influence each other, and the link between them and loneliness is bidirectional, with loneliness often exacerbating the factors that initially placed the older person at risk. Finally, *structural* and *contextual factors* are essential to consider and are depicted in the background of Figure 9–1, including cultural contexts, systemic sources of inequity (including systemic racism and ageism), and access to health care and social resources.

Assessment of loneliness and its contributors is essential to capitalizing on the model we propose. Table 9–1 lists three key resources that can guide a clinician, social service agency, or researcher in selecting the most appropriate assessment tool for loneliness and its contributors for a given subpopulation of older adults and guide the purpose of the assessment (e.g., screening and referral versus treatment outcomes). For health care settings, the report by the National Academies of Sciences, Engineering, and Medicine on addressing social isolation and loneliness in older adults within health care settings may be useful given its focus on challenges and opportunities inherent in these settings. For community agencies, the Campaign to End Loneliness white paper, which includes recommendations for brief screening measures, may be most useful given its focus on practical and brief strategies. Clinicians working with older adults may appreciate the self-assessment tools that can be shared with patients via AARP's Connect2Affect webpages.

In the following sections, we describe the evidence base for programs to address loneliness in older adults, organized by each pathway of our conceptual model. Many interventions could be categorized as useful for a number of pathways to loneliness. In that case, we considered populations in which those interventions have been studied and our own clinical and research experience in working with lonely older adults to guide our synthesis. Table 9–1 includes resources for programs to address loneliness.

Mental Health

Psychotherapeutic Interventions

Two randomized trials with lonely older adults examined brief psychotherapies to reduce loneliness. The first examined an adaptation of behavioral activation—an evidence-based treatment for depression—to address social connection and loneliness in homebound older adults (Pepin et al. 2021). Older adults

TABLE 9–1. Resources for treating loneliness in older adults

Assessment and program planning

AARP's Connect2Affect	https://connect2affect.org/
UK's Campaign to End Loneliness Promising Approaches	www.campaigntoendloneliness.org/ promising-approaches-revisited/
National Academies of Sciences, Engineering, and Medicine's Report on Social Isolation and Loneliness in Older Adults	www.nap.edu/read/25663/chapter/1

Mental health resources: mindfulness and reminiscence

Loving kindness meditations to share with patients	http://headspace.com
Treatment manual and patient workbook for mindfulness exercises	Smart CM: *Wisdom Mind: Mindfulness for Cognitively Healthy Older Adults and Those With Subjective Cognitive Decline.* New York, Oxford University Press, 2021
Birren Center for Autobiographical Studies resources on Guided Autobiography	https://guidedautobiography.com/
Self-guided life review book	Campbell R, Svensson C: *Writing Your Legacy: The Step-by-Step Guide to Crafting Your Life Story.* New York, Writer's Digest Books, 2015
Suggested reminiscence activities for older adults with dementia	www.dementiauk.org/reminiscence-activities/

Socialization and group activities

AARP's Connect2Affect online resources	https://connect2affect.org/
UK's Campaign to End Loneliness suggestions for managing loneliness	www.campaigntoendloneliness.org/ feeling-lonely/
Eldercare locator for aging services across the United States	https://eldercare.acl.gov/
The Institute on Aging's 24-hour toll-free Friendship Line	1-800-971-0016

TABLE 9–1. **Resources for treating loneliness in older adults *(continued)***

Technology

AARP online article and tutorial video for technology	www.aarp.org/home-family/personal-technology/info-2020/how-to-use-zoom.html
Senior Planet pdf tutorial on zoom and practice online events	https://seniorplanet.org/get-involved/online/
Virtual Senior Center	www.vscm.selfhelp.net/

Pets (robotic and real)

Joy for All Pets robotic pets	https://joyforall.com/
Gerontological Society of America resources on Human Animal Interaction	www.geron.org/programs-services/alliances-and-multi-stakeholder-collaborations/human-animal-interaction-and-healthy-aging

Volunteering

AmeriCorps Senior Program	https://americorps.gov/serve/americorps-seniors
Senior Companions	https://americorps.gov/serve/fit-finder/americorps-seniors-senior-companion-program
Foster Grandparents	https://americorps.gov/serve/fit-finder/americorps-seniors-foster-grandparent-program
Retired Senior Volunteer Program (RSVP)	https://americorps.gov/serve/fit-finder/americorps-seniors-rsvp

Connection planning

Worksheets	www.eenet.ca/resource/social-connection-isolated-older-adults
Connections Planning Manual from the VA	www.mirecc.va.gov/visn5/training/connection_plans.asp

receiving Meals on Wheels who reported loneliness were randomly assigned to five weekly sessions of lay-coach-delivered behavioral activation focused on social activities via video call or to five weekly sessions of friendly contacts by video call. Results indicated significantly lower levels of loneliness, increased satisfaction with social support, and increased self-reported social interaction at 6- and 12-week follow-up assessments (Choi et al. 2020). The second study examined an adaptation of Engage Psychotherapy—also an evidence-based treatment for depression in later life—to address social connection and loneliness in older adults at risk for suicide (Van Orden et al. 2021). Primary care patients age 60 and older who endorsed loneliness or feeling like a burden on others were randomly assigned to 10 in-home, face-to-face Engage Psychotherapy sessions focused on social connection (Social Engage) or to care as usual. Results indicated significantly reduced depression symptoms and increased social-emotional quality of life at 10-week follow-up (Van Orden et al. 2021). A study of Engage Psychotherapy for late-life depression found that social activities with another person were the most effective type of activity (vs. pleasant and physical activities) at reducing depression (Solomonov et al. 2019). These studies indicate that brief behavioral therapies hold promise for reducing loneliness and improving depression and quality of life in lonely older adults. Larger samples with more male participants, longer follow-up periods to document the durability of effects, and study of whether changes in loneliness account for longer-term improvements in mood, functioning, and well-being are needed to determine if these programs have enough evidence base for lonely older adults.

Mindfulness Training

One randomized trial with healthy adults ages 55–85 (primarily women) compared 8 weeks of group-delivered mindfulness-based stress reduction (weekly 2-hour group classes, a day-long retreat, 30 minutes at home practice daily) with a waitlist control condition and found significant reductions in levels of loneliness at the end of the program (Creswell et al. 2012). A study with younger and middle-aged adults with elevated stress who received 14 weeks of daily 20-minute audio mindfulness lessons delivered via smartphone (vs. active control training) demonstrated a 22% reduction in loneliness and increased social contact (by two social interactions per day and one additional person per day) (Lindsay et al. 2019), thus quantifying the potential degree of improvements in social behaviors and loneliness that can be expected from mindfulness interventions. Results indicate that mindfulness approaches that teach acceptance and compassion may reduce psychological distress and loneliness in older adults. Future work is needed that enrolls subjects with significant loneliness at baseline and examines the components of mindfulness training that are most useful for loneliness, including loving kindness meditation, which has been shown to increase feelings of social connection (Hutcherson et al. 2008).

Reminiscence and Life Review Programs

Reminiscence programs comprise a range of behavioral interventions, including life review therapy (delivered individually by mental health professionals), life review writing groups, and reminiscence groups. These programs have been found (via meta-analytic review) to improve social integration, which is associated with loneliness, and qualitative analysis of reminiscence provided via groups suggests that feelings of belonging are a key ingredient for improved well-being from participation (Pinquart and Forstmeier 2012). Randomized trials examining loneliness as an outcome have not been conducted. A recent study described a user-centered design process for developing a virtual-reality reminiscence program for older adults with loneliness to help them reconnect with positive memories of others and thereby reframe their current feelings of loneliness within the context of their life stories (Veldmeijer et al. 2020). Reminiscence activities are also useful for older adults with dementia who may not be able to express feelings of loneliness in words but through behaviors such as agitation, confusion, or withdrawal; social connection remains a need for persons with dementia. Reminiscence exercises that allow a caregiver and person with dementia to connect around shared memories and positive experiences can foster social connection between the dyad. Example exercises that can be used are listed in Table 9–1. Results of these studies suggest a potential role for reminiscence programs in a portfolio of programs to reduce loneliness in older adults, with studies needed that focus specifically on loneliness, tease apart the effects due to group participation from reminiscence activities, and determine which subpopulations of older adults might benefit most from such programs.

Socialization and Group Activities

One systematic review of programs to address loneliness and social isolation in older adults concluded that group programs that involve shared interests or provide education and are run by older adults may be effective for reducing loneliness and that these groups may be more effective than one-on-one support programs (Cattan et al. 2005). However, a more recent systematic review did not find evidence that group programs are more effective than one-on-one programs, concluding instead that the common ingredient for effective programs appears to be a focus on activities that provide opportunities for "productive engagement" with others and the community (Gardiner et al. 2018). Examples of productive engagement that may impact feelings of loneliness via group participation include music and art groups (Cohen 2006), educational offerings, and volunteering opportunities.

Physical Health

Wellness and Exercise Classes
for Chronic Conditions

Local agencies on aging (supported by the Older Americans Act) often provide group programming for wellness, managing chronic conditions, falls prevention, and exercise for older adults. Although these programs are not specifically designed to address loneliness, the group format may be both acceptable and provide benefit in terms of loneliness for some older adults, especially in the context of managing chronic conditions. The Leveraging Exercise to Age in Place (LEAP) Study used a non-randomized clinical trial to examine the potential benefits of participation in evidence-based programs commonly offered by aging services agencies for adults ages 50 and older, including "Tai Chi for Arthritis," "Enhance Fitness," and a "Healthier Living Workshop." Results indicated decreased loneliness and increased social support at 6-month follow-up for participants who engaged in at least one program (Mays et al. 2021).

Many programs for social connection and loneliness in older adults are not tailored for racial or ethnic minorities, who may experience unique social stressors and bring unique social strengths to programs. One culturally tailored program for older adults is the Happy Older Latinos are Active (¡HOLA, Amigos!) program, which is a group walking program (45 minutes, three times per week for 16 weeks) that includes a meeting with a community-health worker for older adult (age 60+) Latinx individuals with subthreshold depression/anxiety symptoms. A randomized trial comparing ¡HOLA, Amigos! to a waitlist control condition demonstrated psychosocial benefits, including reduced loneliness (Jimenez et al. 2018). Given that programs marketed as addressing loneliness may be less acceptable to some older adults due to stigma (Kharicha et al. 2017), addressing social connection and loneliness by addressing physical health holds promise.

Social Prescribing

Social prescribing refers to formal referrals by health care providers to non-medical services to address social determinants of health, such as community-based services to reduce social disconnection and loneliness (Hamilton-West et al. 2020). This practice is not new but is gaining greater attention as a possible strategy to address the social needs of older adults. Data directly supporting social prescribing to reduce loneliness for older adults are not available, but available research suggests numerous potential psychosocial benefits when sufficient infrastructure and supports are in place (Alderwick et al. 2018; Woodall et al. 2018). Social prescribing is discussed elsewhere in this book (see Chapter 10, "Community-Based Interventions for Loneliness").

Physical and Cognitive Functional Decline

Home-Delivered Meals and Friendly Calling

Older adults who have physical, cognitive, or sensory impairments may receive home-delivered meals provided by community-based agencies to promote healthy aging and independence. Research suggests such programs offer benefits beyond improved nutrition, with a qualitative analysis of feedback from Meals on Wheels drivers and program staff highlighting the social support component (Thomas et al. 2016). Program evaluations indicate improvements in well-being and loneliness after 2 months of program participation (Wright et al. 2015) but highlight a need for more rigorous study of the psychosocial benefits of home-delivered meals (Campbell et al. 2015).

Friendly calling programs are another service commonly available to homebound older adults. A volunteer-provided friendly calling program (4 weeks of empathy-oriented calls) for Meals on Wheels clients during the COVID-19 pandemic was tested with a randomized trial (care-as-usual comparator) and demonstrated significant effects on loneliness, depressive symptoms, and anxiety symptoms after 4 weeks of calls (Kahlon et al. 2021).

Technology Platforms

For older adults with physical or cognitive limitations that preclude leaving the home, technology platforms have been proposed as a solution for reduced social contact. A meta-analysis of technology interventions to address loneliness in older adults examined interventions that involved computer or internet use to promote psychosocial outcomes and found an overall effect on reduced loneliness, with significant variability between studies and the program studied (Choi et al. 2012). An example of a technology platform designed for older adults to improve social connections is the Personalized Reminder Information and Social Management (PRISM) system, which was developed for community-dwelling older adults at risk for social isolation (Czaja et al. 2015). PRISM involves providing older adults with internet-capable computers that offer several features to promote social connection, including a dynamic classroom feature, email (and PRISM buddy email connections), photos application, games, and a calendar. The intervention also includes online help, an annotated resource guide, three home visits for training, and check-in calls to answer questions and promote uptake. PRISM was tested in a multisite randomized controlled trial and compared with a non-technology control using written resources (plus home visits and check-in calls) (Czaja et al. 2018). The PRISM group reported significantly less loneliness and increased perceived social support and well-being at 6-month follow-up, but these gains were not maintained at 12-month follow-up. Current research on technology platforms for loneliness suggest that these programs likely provide benefit to many older adults, but it is not clear which platforms are most acceptable and accessible to older adults, effective, and affordable.

Pets (Robotic and Real)

Few interventions have been designed to address loneliness specifically for older adults with cognitive impairment. Robotic pets are one such intervention, with various "pets" having been studied, ranging from the FDA-approved PARO seal that provides benefit for older adults with dementia to less expensive dog and cat robotic pets with less sophisticated artificial intelligence. A meta-analysis of robotic pets to improve health and quality of life for older adults included 11 studies and found significant effects on agitation, anxiety, and quality of life, with a potential signal for increased social engagement and reduced loneliness (Pu et al. 2019). Robotic pets have been studied most often in long-term care settings, where congregate living does not necessarily protect against loneliness. One randomized trial that compared a robotic pet group (two times per week) with a care-as-usual condition reported decreased loneliness after 12 weeks, which may be due to increased socialization between residents in the group with the robotic pet (e.g., the pet served as a conversation starter) (Robinson et al. 2013). Research has also examined the benefits of real pets for loneliness in older adults and indicates potential pathways through which pet ownership may mitigate loneliness, including increased physical activity and social interaction, as well as companionship.

Social Function and Social Stressors

Community-Based Services Supported by the Older Americans Act

Local agencies on aging are present throughout the United States and provide a range of non-medical services designed to help older adults maintain independence in their homes. Many (if not all) of the services provided could be conceptualized as programs to reduce loneliness, but few have been examined regarding their benefit for loneliness or social connection. One commonly provided program is *geriatric care management*, but most studies have tested care management provided in health care (e.g., primary care) settings. One randomized controlled trial found improved social functioning for low-income older adults who received 2 years of in-home care management via primary care clinics (Counsell et al. 2007). Senior centers, congregate meals, and support groups are other commonly provided services, but empirical research and program evaluation data are not available to support these programs for reducing loneliness.

Volunteer Opportunities

Volunteer opportunities, including through the national Americorps Senior program, have strong evidence from numerous studies and program evaluations to support benefit for physical health, physical functioning, cognitive functioning, and mental health. However, little work has examined social isolation and loneliness as outcomes despite the promise of such programs to promote meaningful social connection. Evidence is strongest for two AmeriCorps Seniors programs operated by the federal Corporation for National and Community Service, which also operates other national service programs, including AmeriCorps (for younger adults). The Senior Corps is a network of national service programs for Americans age 55 and older and consists of three programs: Senior Companions, Foster Grandparents, and the Retired Senior Volunteer Program (RSVP), all with the objective of improving lives and fostering civic engagement. AmeriCorps Senior programs operate in local communities in all 50 states, the District of Columbia, Puerto Rico, and the Virgin Islands. RSVP volunteers are matched with local volunteer opportunities in their communities based on preferences, skills, and community need. Foster Grandparents are matched with youth and provide mentoring and social support. Senior Companion Program volunteers help older adults maintain independence and remain in their own homes by providing friendly visiting and instrumental support. Foster Grandparent and Senior Companion Program volunteers complete an orientation, receive ongoing support and training, and may be paid a small stipend (for income-eligible volunteers) to help remove the barriers to volunteering and ensure participants do not incur additional costs while serving. Older adults in these programs typically spend 3–4 hours per week volunteering and continue in the program for several years. The Corporation for National and Community Service commissioned an independent evaluation of these programs that describes their benefits to the older volunteers (Georges et al. 2018; Tan et al. 2016). For the Senior Companion Program, most volunteers report high satisfaction with the program because it helped them feel less lonely and more satisfied with their life (Pratt et al. 2014).

Peer Companionship

Peer companionship is a commonly provided program through aging services agencies, including through the AmeriCorps Senior Companions program. The evaluation just mentioned of the benefits of serving as a volunteer also examined the benefits of receiving peer companionship and reported that both the instrumental and supportive functions of peer companionship are described by clients as highly beneficial (Pratt et al. 2014). A randomized trial of peer companionship provided by volunteers (vs. care as usual) in an aging services agency for older adults who reported feeling lonely or like a burden on others found reduced depressive symptoms, anxiety symptoms, and perceptions of being a burden on others after 1 year of the program (Conwell et al. 2021). A qualitative evaluation of a national telephone befriending program in the United Kingdom found that older adults reported feeling like they belonged and were motivated to engage in their community going forward (Cattan et al. 2011). Program evaluation and research data on community programs for older adults suggest that these programs provide a diverse range of benefits to many older adults. Additional study is needed to examine which programs are most effective to reduce or prevent loneliness in older adults, as well as the potential benefits of outreach to older adults who do not actively seek such programs, including through linkages between primary care clinics and community-based programs serving older adults.

Connection Planning

Connection planning is an evidence-informed approach to preventing loneliness in older adults who may be facing life transitions that could impact social connection, such as retirement or relocation to a senior living community. This approach allows older adults to proactively address social connection and potentially prevent loneliness in the context of such transitions. Connection planning can also be used as a brief intervention to reduce loneliness and social isolation. It is a brief behavioral intervention (two 30-minute sessions) that can be either a stand-alone or adjunctive intervention, is intentionally flexible, and can be delivered by mental health professionals or peers. Analogous to safety planning for suicide prevention, connection planning is more intensive than providing simple recommendations for ways to connect; it includes psychoeducation about the importance of being intentional about social connections and relationships and addresses motivational and structural barriers to connecting. It applies a few basic principles from cognitive-behavioral therapy to help older adults improve social connection. The clinician's primary task is assessment, including what is contributing to the older adult's feelings of loneliness, what forms of social connection the person most values, and what barriers exist that make it difficult for the person to connect socially. This assessment helps the clinician tailor the psychoeducation to the thoughts, feelings, and behaviors that may be contributing to the older adult's loneliness and identify three basic interventions that may be useful. Interventions include basic cognitive restructuring around social interactions, relaxation exercises to manage social anxiety, and practical resources for mitigating practical barriers to socialization. Selected strategies are written down on a connections plan for the patient to use in the upcoming weeks, with a planned follow-up check-in by phone to assess progress and any additional barriers that have arisen. Resources for clinicians interested in connection planning appear in Table 9–1.

Community- and Societal-Level Interventions

Our discussion thus far has focused primarily on individual-level risk factors for loneliness and strategies to mitigate those factors. However, loneliness in older adults occurs within communities that can hinder or facilitate meaningful social connection, and thereby these also serve as a target for reducing or preventing loneliness in later life. Societal-level factors that may increase vulnerability to loneliness include systemic racism, ageism, and structural inequalities in access to health care and social resources. Factors such as rurality, socioeconomic status, and access to services are essential to address. The intersection of age-specific risk factors for loneliness with other inequities that increase risk for loneliness will be essential to developing the most effective strategies to address loneliness in later life and at all ages (Robert Wood Johnson Foundation 2020). Most of the programs discussed thus far in this chapter have been tested with white, English-speaking older adults, with little focus on older adults of color or on speakers of languages other than English. Experiences such as linguistic isolation may increase risk for loneliness, whereas community cohesion may mitigate risk. Research is needed on how to optimize programs and community resources to address these factors. Community interventions are discussed in Chapter 10.

One approach is the Age Friendly Community (as termed by the World Health Organization, www.who.int/ageing/age-friendly environments/en). This approach to equity for older adults acknowledges that every older person is embedded in a physical and social environment that can either promote or hinder quality of life and engagement with their community as they age. The World Health Organization maintains an online "Global Database of Age-Friendly Practices" with examples from around the world in numerous domains relevant to social connection and loneliness, including intentional design of outdoor spaces and buildings to promote accessibility for older adults with mobility limitations, transportation infrastructure for older adults unable to drive, and programs to promote and support social participation of individuals of all ages. Addressing ageism is also an essential component of Age Friendly Communities and may include educational campaigns and policies to reduce ageism and acknowledge value of people at all ages.

Case Vignette

George Eastman was born on July 12, 1854, into a family of modest means in rural western New York. Curious and driven to succeed, by the time of his death by suicide in 1932 at the age of 77, his legacy included the multinational Kodak corporation, fabulous wealth, and a record of philanthropy that lives to this day. His suicide note said simply, "My work is done. Why wait?" suggesting satisfaction, autonomy, and self-determination at the end of a life well lived.

In truth, however, the story of Mr. Eastman's final months was one of isolation, loneliness, pain, and demoralization. The reasons for his social isolation and ultimately his death were multiple—the "pathways" to loneliness and despair proposed in this chapter. He was physically ill with a painful, degenerative disease of the spine. His illness left him increasingly debilitated, functionally limited, and restricted to his mansion home. Never having married, he had few family or close friends and had been forced to relinquish his work, the ultimate source of meaning in his life. His stressors were many, and his personal resources diminishing. He was demoralized, and although his social status and cultural mores inhibited discussion of his mental health, he was thought to be depressed and, ultimately, alone and lonely. Suicide, George Eastman believed, was his only option.

Summary

In many ways, the science of promoting social connection in later life is in its infancy. Yet we know a great deal about the power of social connection to promote health and, conversely, the detrimental impact of loneliness on health and well-being. Research and clinical experience clearly document that social connection matters for health, well-being, and longevity in later life; social isolation and loneliness have many causes and consequences in later life; and behavioral interventions can reduce loneliness and social isolation for older adults. It is not clear yet which interventions are most effective, for whom, and in what circumstances nor which mechanisms are essential to achieve positive outcomes. Thus, it is not yet clear which programs are evidence-based for loneliness nor how to tailor intervention strategies to address individualized contributors to loneliness and isolation.

In the absence of clear evidence-based recommendations, our organization of the literature on interventions for loneliness in later life may assist clinicians and others working with older adults in selecting the programs most likely to benefit an older adult given individual contributors to loneliness, preferences, and contextual circumstances. Our synthesis also suggests areas in need of future study. First, numerous programs to address loneliness in later life are available and provided in the community. These programs are indexed and described in several places (Table 9–1), including AARP's Connect2Affect resource list, the United Kingdom's Campaign to End Loneliness summary of promising practices for loneliness in later life, and the report from the National Academies of Sciences, Engineering, and Medicine on social isolation and loneliness in older adults. The evidence base for such programs is limited, and future research on existing programs (vs. developing new programs to study) could provide essential information for community agencies, clinicians, and policymakers in charge of funding decisions. Second, many programs for loneliness are not seen as acceptable by older adults, necessitating research methodologies such as co-design and involvement of older adults in all phases of research, including incorporation of qualitative methods in clinical trials. Third, an understanding of key mechanisms whereby interventions are effective in reducing or preventing loneliness is essential for successful implementation outside research settings and application to populations not specifically studied in prior research. Fourth, research is needed on strategies to best match older adults with programs most likely to benefit them and to understand when less- versus more-intensive interventions are needed. Finally, research is needed to clarify the most acceptable and effective modes of delivery for loneliness interventions. The COVID-19 pandemic highlighted the importance of understanding whether interventions for social connection are effective when delivered via videocall or online (Williams et al. 2021). Future work should continue to investigate advantages and disadvantages of remote versus in-person modes of delivery for programs to address loneliness. The numerous pathways to loneliness in later life produce not only a complex problem but also numerous opportunities for intervention and promotion of social connection and well-being in later life.

KEY POINTS

- Loneliness is a threat to health and well-being, even more so among older adults whose physical, mental, functional, and social comorbidities place them at greater risk for adverse outcomes than in younger people.

- There are multiple "pathways" to loneliness in later life, including mental and physical ill health, social stressors, and functional limitations, as well as cultural and sociopolitical contextual factors.

- Individualized prevention and treatment for loneliness in older adults begin with analysis of what pathways contribute to the individual's social disconnections.

- Evidence from intervention and outcomes research indicates that loneliness is modifiable. It remains unclear, however, which interventions work for which older persons and under what circumstances.

- Further research is needed to clarify the specific mechanisms by which different pathways result in loneliness and, on that basis, the effectiveness of interventions best suited to each older person's needs and preferences.

- Contextual factors that make all older people vulnerable to loneliness must be addressed at a universal level.

Suggested Readings

Cacioppo S, Grippo AJ, London S, et al: Loneliness: clinical import and interventions. Perspect Psychol Sci 10(2):238–249, 2015

Gerst-Emerson K, Jayawardhana J: Loneliness as a public health issue: the impact of loneliness on health care utilization among older adults. Am J Public Health 105(5):1013–1019, 2015

Holt-Lunstad J, Robles TF, Sbarra DA: Advancing social connection as a public health priority in the United States. Am Psychol 72(6):517–530, 2017

Pepin R, Stevens CJ, Choi NG, et al: Modifying behavioral activation to reduce social isolation and loneliness among older adults. Am J Geriatr Psychiatry 29(8):761-770, 2021

Williams CYK, Townson AT, Kapur M, et al: Interventions to reduce social isolation and loneliness during COVID-19 physical distancing measures: a rapid systematic review. PLoS One 16(2):e0247139, 2021

References

Aartsen M, Jylhä M: Onset of loneliness in older adults: results of a 28 year prospective study. Eur J Ageing 8(1):31–38, 2011 21475393

Alderwick HAJ, Gottlieb LM, Fichtenberg CM, Adler NE: Social prescribing in the U.S. and England: emerging interventions to address patients' social needs. Am J Prev Med 54(5):715–718, 2018 29551326

Anderson GO: Loneliness among older adults: a national survey of adults 45+. AARP Research, September 2010. Available at: https://www.aarp.org/research/topics/life/info-2014/loneliness_2010.html. Accessed February 2022.

Blazer D: Social isolation and loneliness in older adults: a mental health/public health challenge. JAMA Psychiatry 77(10):990–991, 2020 32492078

Cacioppo JT, Hawkley LC: Social isolation and health, with an emphasis on underlying mechanisms. Perspect Biol Med 46(3 suppl):S39–S52, 2003 14563073

Cacioppo JT, Hawkley LC, Thisted RA: Perceived social isolation makes me sad: 5-year cross-lagged analyses of loneliness and depressive symptomatology in the Chicago Health, Aging, and Social Relations Study. Psychol Aging 25(2):453–463, 2010 20545429

Cacioppo JT, Cacioppo S, Boomsma DI: Evolutionary mechanisms for loneliness. Cogn Emotion 28(1):3–21, 2014 24067110

Cacioppo S, Grippo AJ, London S, et al: Loneliness: clinical import and interventions. Perspect Psychol Sci 10(2):238–249, 2015 25866548

Campbell AD, Godfryd A, Buys DR, Locher JL: Does participation in home-delivered meals programs improve outcomes for older adults? Results of a systematic review. J Nutr Gerontol Geriatr 34(2):124–167, 2015 26106985

Campbell R, Svensson C: Writing Your Legacy: The Step-by-Step Guide to Crafting Your Life Story. New York, Writer's Digest Books, 2015

Carstensen LL, Turan B, Scheibe S, et al: Emotional experience improves with age: evidence based on over 10 years of experience sampling. Psychol Aging 26(1):21–33, 2011 20973600

Cattan M, White M, Bond J, Learmouth A: Preventing social isolation and loneliness among older people: a systematic review of health promotion interventions. Ageing Soc 25(01):41–67, 2005

Cattan M, Kime N, Bagnall AM: The use of telephone befriending in low level support for socially isolated older people--an evaluation. Health Soc Care Community 19(2):198–206, 2011 21114564

Charles ST, Carstensen LL: Social and emotional aging. Annu Rev Psychol 61:383–409, 2010 19575618

Choi M, Kong S, Jung D: Computer and internet interventions for loneliness and depression in older adults: a meta-analysis. Healthc Inform Res 18(3):191–198, 2012 23115742

Choi NG, Pepin R, Marti CN, et al: Improving social connectedness for homebound older adults: randomized controlled trial of tele-delivered behavioral activation versus tele-delivered friendly visits. Am J Geriatr Psychiatry 28(7):698–708, 2020 32238297

Cohen GD: Research on creativity and aging: the positive impact of the arts on health and illness. Generations 30:7–15, 2006

Cohen S, Janicki-Deverts D: Can we improve our physical health by altering our social networks? Perspect Psychol Sci 4(4):375–378, 2009 20161087

Cohen-Mansfield J, Perach R: Interventions for alleviating loneliness among older persons: a critical review. Am J Health Promot 29(3):e109–e125, 2015 24575725

Cohen-Mansfield J, Hazan H, Lerman Y, Shalom V: Correlates and predictors of loneliness in older-adults: a review of quantitative results informed by qualitative insights. Int Psychogeriatr 28(4):557–576, 2016 26424033

Conwell Y, Van Orden KA, Stone DM, et al: Peer companionship for mental health of older adults in primary care: a pragmatic, nonblinded, parallel-group, randomized controlled trial. Am J Geriatr Psychiatry 29(8):748–757, 2021 (2020)

Counsell SR, Callahan CM, Clark DO, et al: Geriatric care management for low-income seniors: a randomized controlled trial. JAMA 298(22):2623–2633, 2007 18073358

Creswell JD, Irwin MR, Burklund LJ, et al: Mindfulness-based stress reduction training reduces loneliness and pro-inflammatory gene expression in older adults: a small randomized controlled trial. Brain Behav Immun 26(7):1095–1101, 2012 22820409

Czaja SJ, Boot WR, Charness N, et al: The Personalized Reminder Information and Social Management system (PRISM) trial: rationale, methods and baseline characteristics. Contemp Clin Trials 40:35–46, 2015 25460342

Czaja SJ, Boot WR, Charness N, et al: Improving social support for older adults through technology: findings from the PRISM randomized controlled trial. Gerontologist 58(3):467–477, 2018

Dickens AP, Richards SH, Greaves CJ, Campbell JL: Interventions targeting social isolation in older people: a systematic review. BMC Public Health 11:647, 2011 21843337

Findlay RA: Interventions to reduce social isolation amongst older people: where is the evidence? Ageing Soc 23(5):647–658, 2003

Gardiner C, Geldenhuys G, Gott M: Interventions to reduce social isolation and loneliness among older people: an integrative review. Health Soc Care Community 26(2):147–157, 2018 27413007

Georges A, Fung W, Smith J, et al: Longitudinal Study of Foster Grandparent and Senior Companion Programs: Service Delivery Implications and Health Benefits to the Volunteers. North Bethesda, MD, JBS International, 2018

Gerst-Emerson K, Jayawardhana J: Loneliness as a public health issue: the impact of loneliness on health care utilization among older adults. Am J Public Health 105(5):1013–1019, 2015 25790413

Golden J, Conroy RM, Bruce I, et al: Loneliness, social support networks, mood and wellbeing in community-dwelling elderly. Int J Geriatr Psychiatry 24(7):694–700, 2009 19274642

Hagan R, Manktelow R, Taylor BJ, Mallett J: Reducing loneliness amongst older people: a systematic search and narrative review. Aging Ment Health 18(6):683–693, 2014 24437736

Hamilton-West K, Milne A, Hotham S: New horizons in supporting older people's health and wellbeing: is social prescribing a way forward? Age Ageing 49(3):319–326, 2020 32080727

Hawkley LC, Thisted RA, Cacioppo JT: Loneliness predicts reduced physical activity: cross-sectional & longitudinal analyses. Health Psychol 28(3):354–363, 2009 19450042

Hawkley LC, Thisted RA, Masi CM, Cacioppo JT: Loneliness predicts increased blood pressure: 5-year cross-lagged analyses in middle-aged and older adults. Psychol Aging 25(1):132–141, 2010 20230134

Heikkinen RL, Kauppinen M: Mental well-being: a 16-year follow-up among older residents in Jyväskylä. Arch Gerontol Geriatr 52(1):33–39, 2011 20207429

Holmén K, Furukawa H: Loneliness, health and social network among elderly people: a follow-up study. Arch Gerontol Geriatr 35(3):261–274, 2002 14764365

Holt-Lunstad J: Loneliness and social isolation as risk factors: the power of social connection in prevention. Am J Lifestyle Med 15(5):567–573, 2021 34646109

Holt-Lunstad J, Smith TB, Layton JB: Social relationships and mortality risk: a meta-analytic review. PLoS Med 7(7):e1000316, 2010 20668659

Holt-Lunstad J, Robles TF, Sbarra DA: Advancing social connection as a public health priority in the United States. Am Psychol 72(6):517–530, 2017 28880099

Holwerda TJ, Deeg DJ, Beekman A, et al: Feelings of loneliness, but not social isolation, predict dementia onset: results from the Amsterdam Study of the Elderly (AMSTEL). J Neurol Neurosurg Psychiatry 85(2):135–142, 2014

Hoogendijk EO, Suanet B, Dent E, et al: Adverse effects of frailty on social functioning in older adults: results from the Longitudinal Aging Study Amsterdam. Maturitas 83:45–50, 2016 26428078

Huber M, Knottnerus JA, Green L, et al: How should we define health? BMJ 343:d4163, 2011 21791490

Hutcherson CA, Seppala EM, Gross JJ: Loving-kindness meditation increases social connectedness. Emotion 8(5):720–724, 2008 18837623

Jimenez DE, Syed S, Perdomo-Johnson D, Signorile JF: ¡HOLA, amigos! Toward preventing anxiety and depression in older Latinos. Am J Geriatr Psychiatry 26(2):250–256, 2018 28760514

Jylhä M: Old age and loneliness: cross-sectional and longitudinal analyses in the Tampere Longitudinal Study on Aging. Can J Aging 23(2):157–168, 2004 15334815

Kahlon MK, Aksan N, Aubrey R, et al: Effect of layperson-delivered, empathy-focused program of telephone calls on loneliness, depression, and anxiety among adults during the COVID-19 pandemic: a randomized clinical trial. JAMA Psychiatry 78(6):616–622, 2021 33620417

Kharicha K, Iliffe S, Manthorpe J, et al: What do older people experiencing loneliness think about primary care or community based interventions to reduce loneliness? A qualitative study in England. Health Soc Care Community 25(6):1733–1742, 2017 28231615

Kinsella K, Wan H: An Aging World: 2008. Washington, DC, U.S. Census Bureau, 2009

Lindsay EK, Young S, Brown KW, et al: Mindfulness training reduces loneliness and increases social contact in a randomized controlled trial. Proc Natl Acad Sci USA 116(9):3488–3493, 2019 30808743

Luo Y, Hawkley LC, Waite LJ, Cacioppo JT: Loneliness, health, and mortality in old age: a national longitudinal study. Soc Sci Med 74(6):907–914, 2012 22326307

Masi CM, Chen HY, Hawkley LC, Cacioppo JT: A meta-analysis of interventions to reduce loneliness. Pers Soc Psychol Rev 15(3):219–266, 2011 20716644

Mays AM, Kim S, Rosales K, et al: The Leveraging Exercise to Age in Place (LEAP) study: engaging older adults in community-based exercise classes to impact loneliness and social isolation. Am J Geriatr Psychiatry 29(8):777–788, 2021 33268235

O'Rourke HM, Collins L, Sidani S: Interventions to address social connectedness and loneliness for older adults: a scoping review. BMC Geriatr 18(1):214, 2018 30219034

Pepin R, Stevens CJ, Choi NG, et al: Modifying behavioral activation to reduce social isolation and loneliness among older adults. Am J Geriatr Psychiatry 29(8):761–770, 2021 32980253

Perissinotto CM, Stijacic Cenzer I, Covinsky KE: Loneliness in older persons: a predictor of functional decline and death. Arch Intern Med 172(14):1078–1083, 2012 22710744

Pinquart M, Forstmeier S: Effects of reminiscence interventions on psychosocial outcomes: a meta-analysis. Aging Ment Health 16(5):541–558, 2012 22304736

Pratt D, Lovegrove P, Birmingham C, et al: Senior Companion Program Independent Living Performance Measurement Survey: Process, Rationale, Results, and Recommendations. North Bethesda, MD, JBS International, 2014

Preece DA, Goldenberg A, Becerra R, et al: Loneliness and emotion regulation. Pers Individ Dif 180:110974, 2021

Pu L, Moyle W, Jones C, Todorovic M: The effectiveness of social robots for older adults: a systematic review and meta-analysis of randomized controlled studies. Gerontologist 59(1):e37–e51, 2019 29897445

Qualter P, Vanhalst J, Harris R, et al: Loneliness across the life span. Perspect Psychol Sci 10(2):250–264, 2015 25910393

Robert Wood Johnson Foundation: Solutions for social isolation: what we can learn from the world. Coronavirus Pandemic (COVID-19): An RWJF Collection, August 10, 2020. Available at: https://www.rwjf.org/en/library/research/2020/08/solutions-for-social-isolation--what-we-can-learn-from-the-world.html. Accessed February 2022.

Robinson H, Macdonald B, Kerse N, Broadbent E: The psychosocial effects of a companion robot: a randomized controlled trial. J Am Med Dir Assoc 14(9):661–667, 2013 23545466

Rubenowitz E, Waern M, Wilhelmson K, Allebeck P: Life events and psychosocial factors in elderly suicides: a case-control study. Psychol Med 31(7):1193–1202, 2001 11681545

Sabir M, Wethington E, Breckman R, et al: A community-based participatory critique of social isolation intervention research for community-dwelling older adults. J Appl Gerontol 28(2):218–234, 2009 25165409

Scheibe S, Carstensen LL: Emotional aging: recent findings and future trends. J Gerontol B Psychol Sci Soc Sci 65B(2):135–144, 2010 20054013

Shankar A, McMunn A, Banks J, Steptoe A: Loneliness, social isolation, and behavioral and biological health indicators in older adults. Health Psychol 30(4):377–385, 2011 21534675

Solomonov N, Bress JN, Sirey JA, et al: Engagement in socially and interpersonally rewarding activities as a predictor of outcome in "Engage" behavioral activation therapy for late-life depression. Am J Geriatr Psychiatry 27(6):571–578, 2019 30797650

Steptoe A, Shankar A, Demakakos P, Wardle J: Social isolation, loneliness, and all-cause mortality in older men and women. Proc Natl Acad Sci USA 110(15):5797–5801, 2013 23530191

Stuart A, Stevenson C, Koschate M, et al: "Oh no, not a group!" The factors that lonely or isolated people report as barriers to joining groups for health and well-being. Br J Health Psychol 27(1):179–193, 2022 34028949

Tan EJ, Georges A, Gabbard SM, et al: The 2013–2014 Senior Corps Study: foster grandparents and senior companions. Public Policy Aging Rep 26(3):88–95, 2016

Theeke LA: Sociodemographic and health-related risks for loneliness and outcome differences by loneliness status in a sample of U.S. older adults. Res Gerontol Nurs 3(2):113–125, 2010 20415360

Thomas KS, Akobundu U, Dosa D: More than a meal? A randomized control trial comparing the effects of home-delivered meals programs on participants' feelings of loneliness. J Gerontol B Psychol Sci Soc Sci 71(6):1049–1058, 2016

Tomaka J, Thompson S, Palacios R: The relation of social isolation, loneliness, and social support to disease outcomes among the elderly. J Aging Health 18(3):359–384, 2006 16648391

U.N. Department of Economic and Social Affairs: World Population Prospects 2019: Highlights (ST/ESA/SER.A/423). New York, U.N. Department of Economic and Social Affairs, Population Division, 2019

United Nations: World Population Prospects: The 2008 Revision. New York, United Nations, 2009

Van Orden KA, Areán PA, Conwell Y: A pilot randomized trial of engage psychotherapy to increase social connection and reduce suicide risk in later life. Am J Geriatr Psychiatry 29(8):789–800, 2021 33952416

Veldmeijer L, Wartena B, Terlouw G, van't Veer J: Reframing loneliness through the design of a virtual reality reminiscence artefact for older adults. Design Health (Abingdon) 4(3):407–426, 2020

Victor CR, Bowling A: A longitudinal analysis of loneliness among older people in Great Britain. J Psychol 146(3):313–331, 2012 22574423

Waern M, Rubenowitz E, Wilhelmson K: Predictors of suicide in the old elderly. Gerontology 49(5):328–334, 2003 12920354

Weiss RS: Loneliness: The Experience of Emotional and Social Isolation. Cambridge, MA, MIT Press, 1973

Wenger GC, Burholt V: Changes in levels of social isolation and loneliness among older people in a rural area: a twenty-year longitudinal study. Can J Aging 23(2):115–127, 2004 15334812

Whisman MA: Loneliness and the metabolic syndrome in a population-based sample of middle-aged and older adults. Health Psychol 29(5):550–554, 2010 20836610

Williams CYK, Townson AT, Kapur M, et al: Interventions to reduce social isolation and loneliness during COVID-19 physical distancing measures: a rapid systematic review. PLoS One 16(2):e0247139, 2021 33596273

Woodall J, Trigwell J, Bunyan AM, et al: Understanding the effectiveness and mechanisms of a social prescribing service: a mixed method analysis. BMC Health Serv Res 18(1):604, 2018 30081874

Wright L, Vance L, Sudduth C, Epps JB: The impact of a home-delivered meal program on nutritional risk, dietary intake, food security, loneliness, and social well-being. J Nutr Gerontol Geriatr 34(2):218–227, 2015 26106989

10

Community-Based Interventions for Loneliness

Phaedra Bell, Ph.D.
Brian Lawlor, M.D.

> What should young people do with their lives today?
> Many things obviously. But the most daring thing is
> to create stable communities in which the terrible
> disease of loneliness can be cured.
>
> *Kurt Vonnegut*

LONELINESS, the subjective and painful experience of being dissatisfied with one's social relationships, is a common experience across the life span. Although universally experienced in transient forms, persistent loneliness is associated with poor health outcomes, including higher rates of depression, anxiety, and suicide. While loneliness has a similar level of impact on health as smoking and a greater impact than hypertension and obesity, it has failed to rise to the level of a public health focus in most countries. There is a growing awareness among policymakers of the public health importance of loneliness, but robust evidence for effective interventions to decrease loneliness at a community level is still lacking.

Social isolation is a more objectively defined term that corresponds to the frequency and number of a person's social contacts and social network size. Although loneliness and isolation are distinct entities, they often occur together, and isolation is a risk factor for loneliness. Isolation is associated with poor health outcomes on its own, and it is difficult to characterize the independent contributions of isolation and loneliness based on the methodology of studies that have reported the health impacts of both loneliness and isolation to date (Valtorta et al. 2016).

In the design and implementation of community interventions, it is important to distinguish whether loneliness, isolation, or both are being targeted. Individuals who are isolated and not particularly lonely will likely benefit from different approaches than those who are lonely but not isolated (McHugh et al. 2017). Varying combinations of social isolation and loneliness may pose different levels of risk and require customized approaches.

This chapter summarizes existing approaches to reduce loneliness at a population and community level from a number of countries, reviews the evidence for what is effective, describes the evidence gaps, and presents what is needed to advance community-based programs as advocated by Vonnegut (1981).

A Threat to Public Health?

Loneliness is believed by many experts to be a significant threat to public health. Loneliness meets many of the criteria for identifying important public health issues: the size and seriousness of the problem, the economic and social impact at societal and individual levels, inequity in how it affects different groups, and the potential to intervene and prevent it (Table 10–1) (Centers for Disease Control and Prevention 2013).

In the United Kingdom, chronic loneliness affects between 10% and 15% of the population, varying by age group (Jopling and Sserwanja 2016), and significantly impacts health and mortality (O'Luanaigh and Lawlor 2008). In the United States, Australia, and many European countries, loneliness is consistently associated with increased doctor visits in all age groups (Kung et al. 2021), with estimates of $7 billion in extra costs due to additional doctor visits, increased health care utilization, and loss of work productivity (Burns et al. 2022; Gerst-Emerson and Jayawardhana 2015). A U.K. study estimated the total cost to employers, including absenteeism, caring, lost productivity, and turnover, from loneliness experienced by their employees to be £2.5 billion per year (Michaelson et al. 2017). Over a 10-year period, the costs of loneliness to health and social care services were estimated to be more than £6,000 per person for older people suffering most severely from loneliness (McDaid et al. 2017).

TABLE 10–1. Identifying loneliness as a public health priority

Criterion	Evidence
Size and seriousness (disease burden)	Loneliness affects a significant proportion of the population regardless of age group and has increased during the COVID-19 pandemic. It will likely increase further given the global aging populations. Persistent loneliness is associated with increased all-cause mortality, increased depression, and lower quality of life.
Economic and social impact	Costs are increased significantly due to health effects, excess doctor visits, and increased health care utilization
Potential to intervene and prevent	Prevention of loneliness in the general population and intervention for at-risk groups and those with loneliness are possible. Challenges arise with the efficacy, cost-effectiveness, and implementation of interventions at a community level. Successful implementation requires significant cooperation between voluntary and statutory sectors.
Preventive strategies not in place	The evidence base for prevention and interventions is limited, and few countries have identified loneliness as a public health issue.
Inequities	Loneliness disproportionately affects the socially disadvantaged, the poor, and those with preexisting mental health conditions and poor physical health.
International significance	Loneliness increasingly has been recognized as an important public health problem, although data and research relating to its health impact come primarily from high-income countries.
Political will to address the issue	Political will has been variable in the past, but the COVID-19 pandemic has raised awareness of the impact of social isolation and loneliness on mental and physical health that may lead to stronger public, professional, and political engagement.

Some individuals who are lonely and isolated see their doctors not only for medical reasons but also for social connection with someone they trust. *Social prescribing* is a practice developed in the United Kingdom in which physicians and other primary care providers refer patients to a range of non-clinical local services. This practice has emerged as a means to enhance social connection in isolated or lonely individuals who present to health care providers.

There is also evidence of decreased utilization of health care, including preventative health services, in other socially isolated and lonely individuals. It is difficult to specify the independent cost contributions of loneliness and social isolation to total costs of care and what can be saved by addressing loneliness alone, given the frequent co-occurrence of loneliness and social isolation and their overlapping effects on health conditions, particularly mental illness. To date, there is limited research on the distinct economic impacts of loneliness and interventions.

Regarding the potential to intervene and the availability of treatments, it is debatable whether loneliness meets this criterion based on available evidence-based interventions. A National Academies of Sciences, Engineering, and Medicine (2020) report indicated few proven interventions to reduce loneliness and isolation. In general, the evidence base for interventions in loneliness is characterized by small trials lacking a strong theoretical framework and methodology. Community intervention programs, where they exist, also lack robust empirical evidence (Fried et al. 2020).

Several countries, including the United Kingdom and Australia, have been proactive in addressing loneliness at a public health level despite the limited evidence for effective interventions. The United Kingdom launched its first Loneliness Strategy in 2018 in England, building on the work of national and community organizations working in this area (HM Government 2018). In fact, the United Kingdom and, more recently, Japan have appointed a "minister for loneliness" because of the breadth and seriousness of the public health threat posed by loneliness, including increased depression and suicide rates in older people attributable to loneliness.

However, most countries have not recognized or prioritized loneliness as a major threat to the health and well-being of their populations despite the strong evidence for its negative impact on health. This may be partly because loneliness is not accepted as a serious health issue or disease and has previously been viewed as a normal part of growing older. Variability in reported prevalence and incidence due to differences in definitions of social connection and in measurement tools and the lack of a robust evidence base for effective interventions (Prohaska et al. 2020) may have contributed to the slow recognition of loneliness as a critical public health issue.

Tackling Loneliness at the Public Health Level

Public health approaches include increasing awareness through information campaigns and addressing risk factors at individual and population levels.

There is broad agreement about the need to build coalitions across services and sectors, such as transportation to facilitate access to activities and housing to promote interaction and community. These structural components can be as important as community services and other supports. Approaches adopted in the United Kingdom, Australia, and Japan can help inform policy and practice in other countries. In the United Kingdom, The Campaign to End Loneliness (www.campaigntoendloneliness.org) has developed categories of interventions, including information and signposting (i.e., the practice of directing a person toward the right service for their situation), support for individuals, group interventions, awareness and health promotion, and creating broader community engagement, that could be effective in addressing loneliness (Bolton 2012; Jopling 2015). The latest version of their Promising Approaches Framework identifies four major approaches: connector services, gateway infrastructure, direct solutions, and systems-level approaches. Connector services help identify lonely individuals in communities so that they can participate in direct solutions, such as individual and group interventions. Gateway infrastructure includes transportation, digital access, and a built environment that can either facilitate or impede access to direct solutions. Systems-level approaches leverage local assets, such as volunteers or community-based organizations, to support and develop the connector, gateway, and connector approaches. Although more robust evidence is needed to support the effectiveness of these approaches, experience from this campaign has revealed important principles, including the importance of flexibility, of taking an individualized approach to interventions, and of ensuring, as much as possible, the active engagement of stakeholders in the co-creation and co-production of interventions.

In Japan, a super-aging society, there have been significant challenges in dealing with isolation and loneliness in older people. One popular model in both Japan and the United Kingdom has emphasized collaboration between local governments, older citizens, and community groups in the design of interventions. In many instances, this has resulted in the creation of community cafes where older people gather for activities. Older residents report improvement in happiness, but the effectiveness of these co-produced local community solutions has not yet been robustly evaluated (Suzuki et al. 2021).

In Australia, federal, state, and local governments have provided various systems of support to address loneliness and social isolation. The National Community Visitors Scheme funds community volunteers to visit older people who are lonely and isolated. More recently, a coalition of organizations called Ending Loneliness Together is working to break down silos of

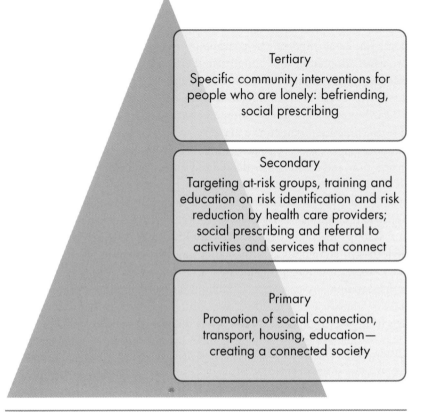

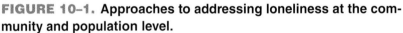

FIGURE 10–1. Approaches to addressing loneliness at the community and population level.

activity and involve diverse community stakeholders at all levels to inform a national strategy. Although increasingly recognized as an important public health issue in Australia, there is no national plan or strategy in place as yet.

Community Approaches to Loneliness

At the community level, there are multilevel approaches to both the prevention and treatment of loneliness (Figure 10–1).

Primary Prevention Approaches

Access to and availability of community activities within a more prosocial, connected society will indirectly decrease loneliness and support people at risk. Many of the root causes of loneliness are structural and socially determined. The availability of high-quality physical and mental health care will decrease disability, improve autonomy, and thereby indirectly decrease the risk of isolation and loneliness. Easy access to transportation and to age-friendly planning and design of neighborhood environments will facilitate social connection. All sectors of society, including health, transportation, housing, employment, education, environment, and food and nutrition, are relevant to preventing loneliness and providing supports for those who are lonely or at risk. For these reasons, a networked and connected sector-wide approach is necessary to tackle the environmental and structural issues that affect the base level of loneliness in the community.

Health promotion efforts that directly target social connection and emphasize the health benefits of maintaining social relationships is another important strategy to decrease loneliness across the life span. This approach should begin at a very early stage and should be promoted as a health value in schools and at every opportunity across the life cycle. Increasingly, the benefits of social connection for health, and particularly brain health, are being actively promoted, although more needs to be done at a policy and public health level.

Secondary and Tertiary Prevention

Direct community interventions can decrease loneliness in those who are lonely and those at-risk. These include targeted, one-to-one befriending schemes, social group services, and support (or link) workers who identify lonely and difficult-to-reach individuals and deliver emotional, practical, and social support and referral to appropriate local services. Social prescribing and peer-to-peer befriending programs are good examples of this type of approach.

Identifying individuals at risk of loneliness requires education efforts targeted at health care professionals, particularly primary care physicians. The importance of loneliness to health and how to ask about it have not been traditional parts of medical school education and clinical training. Screening patients for loneliness and other aspects of social connection at each doctor visit is just as important as measuring their blood pressure and other vital signs.

Community Interventions

General Principles for Effective Interventions

Although the evidence base for the efficacy of community interventions for loneliness is relatively weak, several general principles arise from the literature that, if adopted, point to a greater likelihood of success for a particular intervention. For example, interventions that are peer led and link the person back into their own community may be more likely to show a reduction in loneliness. Regarding approaches to increase social interaction, social facilitation interventions with existing peers and social networks may be more beneficial than trying to encourage new friendships (Williams et al. 2021). Interventions that are participative and actively engage the older person in co-creation or co-production also may work better (Dickens et al. 2011). Although group interventions for loneliness were originally thought to be more effective (Cattan et al. 2005), one-to-one peer support and befriending interventions may also be successful (Lawlor et al. 2014). Taking an individualized approach and training volunteers and facilitators appear to be important factors that can promote success of the intervention.

Social Prescribing

Social prescribing is a form of community intervention that connects formal health care systems with local organizations and services that promote social connection. People attending primary or secondary care services for non-medical reasons can be referred and connected to resources and supports within their own community to improve their health and well-being. Social prescribing is increasingly used as a response to loneliness and isolation identified in older people during health care encounters. It has become one of the cornerstones of the current U.K. public health strategy to combat loneliness and an important component of the *NHS Long-Term Plan* (National Health Service 2019). There are several different models for social prescribing, but most center around a "link worker," someone who can connect an individual to community support services and resources (Kilgarriff-Foster and O'Cathain 2015; Polley et al. 2017). Link workers usually have an in-depth knowledge of community services within a particular area, and their role is to connect individuals to these community resources after referral from a health care professional. Evidence broadly supports the effectiveness of social prescribing for reducing demands in primary care, but the quality of this evidence is relatively weak (Bickerdike et al. 2017). The rationale for social prescribing is that it allows primary care physicians to refer patients with loneliness, or those at risk of loneliness, for tailored services to support their level of social connection, health, and well-being. From a theoretical perspective, facilitating the connection to the patient's own community and thereby strengthening the patient's sense of group identity may be a key component to reducing certain types of loneliness (Jetten et al. 2017).

There is growing evidence that social prescribing can reduce loneliness (Foster et al. 2021; Holding et al. 2020) and improve quality of life in people who were lonely and at risk of loneliness. Foster et al. (2021) found that having skilled link workers and support tailored to the individual were key to a successful intervention. In their study, people younger than 50 years showed the greatest reduction in loneliness. This finding directly challenges the stereotype that older people are more lonely and in greater need of interventions. It also points to the possibility that younger people have greater social loneliness that can be addressed by social prescribing, whereas older people may have greater emotional loneliness due to bereavement that is less amenable to this type of intervention.

Social prescribing to enhance connection and activities can be effective for many people, but some individuals' hypervigilance and mistrust due to loneliness will require referral to community programs or services in which skill-building and a more therapeutic or supportive approach are available. A major function of social prescribing by the link worker is "signposting," or directing the person with loneliness to the appropriate service in the community. However, some communities may have a dearth of accessible services, particularly for older men. Keeping the person connected to a service or activity in a sustainable way can be another challenge. Social prescribing offers major advantages as a means to directly tackle loneliness by identifying people at risk, intervening early, and building networks of people across sectors (e.g., health care, social care, transport). More funding to establish community resources, to train and educate health care professionals, and to evaluate services is essential to effectively integrate social prescribing more broadly into the health and social care systems.

Digital technology holds promise for amplifying social prescribing by overcoming barriers to participation, such as mobility or transportation limitations. However, people who are lonely, especially older people, may also lack computer literacy or access to technology. To remedy these inequities, personnel and programs addressing digital education and access to affordable technology must be incorporated into the design and implementation of community interventions.

Peer Befriending to Reduce Loneliness

In an early review, befriending and home visiting programs were not found to be effective in reducing loneliness, although qualitative research has suggested that these programs can be highly valued, instill greater confidence, and increase community engagement (Cattan et al. 2005; Cattan et al. 2011). It has been proposed that interventions involving peer relationships may be particularly advantageous for sharing common interests and promoting a sense of identity and belonging. There is particular interest in volunteer peer be-friending programs as a scalable community-based response to loneliness.

A pilot randomized controlled trial examined a peer volunteer interven-tion comprising weekly 1-hour visits for 10 weeks over 3 months and found reductions in loneliness and depression in the intervention group compared with treatment as usual at 1 and 3 months following the intervention (Law-lor et al. 2014). The results of this study suggest that peer visits to people who are lonely or at risk of loneliness can maintain benefits beyond the pe-riod of intervention. Qualitative analysis indicated that a key component of a successful outcome was establishing friendship with the volunteer, and many participants planned to keep in touch after the study ended. More than three-quarters of participants reported that the intervention brought positive changes to their lives. A similar study involving older Chinese im-migrants in Canada also showed a significant decrease in loneliness and an increase in resilience in individuals who received weekly peer support and phone calls over a period of 8 weeks (Lai et al. 2020).

Peer volunteer interventions in the community can benefit those who are lonely and those at risk of loneliness and may also benefit the well-being, mood, and feelings of loneliness in volunteers. An improvement in loneli-ness in volunteers delivering peer interventions has been reported in several studies (Carr et al. 2018; Lawlor et al. 2014), and becoming a volunteer has been associated with a decrease in loneliness in those who have been re-cently widowed (Carr et al. 2018). These findings point to volunteering as a potential approach to the prevention or mitigation of loneliness in late life for both volunteers and recipients.

Telephone Support

Peer telephone support may be effective in reducing the experience of lone-liness and social isolation (Cattan et al. 2011). Peer and volunteer "warm lines" that provide a means of connection for lonely people are widely avail-able. They are now being adopted by some private insurance companies in the United States, an acknowledgment of the important health care utiliza-tion and cost implications of loneliness. One such example is Humana and the Institute on Aging Friendship Line, a support line for isolated older adult members. A recent randomized controlled trial during the SARS-CoV-2 (COVID-19) pandemic demonstrated that layperson-delivered empathy-oriented telephone calls resulted in a significant reduction in loneliness, anx-iety, and depression within 4 weeks (Kahlon et al. 2021). An advantage of this study design was the use of lay telephone support workers who received minimal training. Telephone or tele-video interventions delivered by trained lay people may be a cost-effective and scalable approach to addressing loneliness, but the short- and long-term effects of these interventions require more evidence from larger controlled trials.

Video Call Support

The COVID-19 pandemic led to increased use of video calls to connect people at home and at work. A pre-pandemic Cochrane Review evaluated a small number of randomized controlled trials using video calls to reduce social isolation and loneliness in an older adult sample and found no evidence of benefit over care as usual (Noone et al. 2020). A large study of the effects of COVID-19 home confinement in Italy and the Netherlands found that individuals experiencing loneliness were more likely to adopt digital technology to enhance psychosocial support (Bastoni et al. 2021). There was an increase in both the use of and satisfaction from video-calling during the pandemic, pointing to its adaptability and potential long-term benefits for social connection.

Intergenerational Approaches for Loneliness

Intergenerational programs create activities that leverage cooperation, interaction, or exchange between any two generations and usually involve sharing skills or knowledge around an activity. For example, some community programs offer children or young adults the opportunity to learn from the lived experience of the older person and offer the older person a social role, social connection, and a sense of purpose. Two short-term intergenerational community programs specifically examined loneliness as an outcome, with mixed results. One study of older adults and college students found no effect on loneliness (Au et al. 2015), and a second study of older adults and primary school children reported a significant decrease in loneliness (Gaggioli et al. 2014).

The Experience Corps is another example of an intergenerational program that has been reported to improve social connection in older volunteers. Originally developed in 2004 by Linda Fried in Baltimore, Maryland, it was subsequently scaled and expanded across the United States by the AARP. The Experience Corps engages older people from low socioeconomic communities to engage supportively with local elementary students in kindergarten to third grade to help with their reading. In a pilot randomized controlled study, students' reading scores improved, and older volunteers had documented health benefits, including improved physical activity and social activity, compared with control subjects (Fried et al. 2004).

The Multimodal Intergenerational Social Contact Intervention (MISCI) is a San Francisco, California-based program that tackles loneliness by connecting a triad of one lonely older person with two younger partners (Bell et al. 2018). These triads hold regular structured meetings to develop a creative project together over the course of 10 weeks. At the end of 10 weeks, 5–15 triads gather to share their projects. This approach builds on prior evidence that group interventions can have a greater impact on loneliness, and it expands from a dyadic model to triadic model. Keeping the foundational group small allows triads to meet in the homes of the older participants, such as single-occupancy residences, when public health guidelines allow; this accounts for many of the challenges faced by lonely older adults, including mobility limitations, poor transportation infrastructure, or social anxiety, that make it difficult for them to leave their home. The final gathering of triads, supported by special transport and now trusted younger partners, allows the older members to try participation in a larger-group setting with more social scaffolding. Preliminary data from the evaluation of MISCI indicate that it is effective in decreasing loneliness in older participants (Bell et al. 2019).

Intergenerational programs hold promise as useful community interventions to enhance social connection, particularly for older people, but these programs must be evaluated more rigorously with larger numbers and using high-quality evaluative design and methodology (Jarrott et al. 2022). As with all community interventions for loneliness, longer-term evaluation of outcomes and cost-effectiveness—beyond the short duration of the intervention—is also required.

Use of Technology

During the COVID-19 pandemic, use of technology to connect people to support systems, family, and health and social services became accelerated. Research on the use of the internet to improve connection and decrease loneliness has been limited; many of the studies have lacked methodological rigor, and results have been mixed (Casanova et al. 2021). A recent study reviewed pre-COVID-19 experimental studies using training in information and communication technologies, such as personal computers, laptops, smartphones, tablets with email and the internet, and social networking sites to improve levels of well-being or loneliness in older adults. Eleven studies and 953 participants met inclusion criteria. Studies noted improvements in loneliness and other well-being aspects such as sense of self-worth, strength of personal identity, and self-esteem.

In a separate randomized trial, a specifically designed computer system, the Personal Reminder Information and Social Management (PRISM) system, was studied in 300 older adults. Those trained in PRISM had less loneliness and greater perceived social support and well-being compared with a control condition at 6 months (Czaja et al. 2018). This system included instructor support and a user-centered design that may have been important features to promote success. Although these results are promising, further research with large randomized controlled trials is needed to fully support the use of information and communication technologies to decrease loneliness (Casanova et al. 2021).

Case Vignette

At a routine visit, John, a 67-year-old man informed his primary care provider that he had been feeling increasingly lonely and sad since his retirement at age 65. The physician suggested participating in a program with group activities at the local community center that included organized trips for retired people. John explained that he was trying to make himself participate in these opportunities but that he was forgetful with names and was worried about embarrassing or humiliating himself in social situations. When the physician referred John to a psychiatrist, she assessed him for both his memory complaints and his emotional symptoms. She found that he had subjective memory concerns (but no objective deficits), depression, anxiety, and loneliness and diagnosed him with clinically significant depression and anxiety. She prescribed a selective serotonin reuptake inhibitor antidepressant.

At follow-up, John reported that his mood had improved, but he still felt lonely and lacked confidence to engage with opportunities in the community. The psychiatrist referred him to a befriending program that sent volunteers to visit lonely and isolated older people in his community, but after several months, he continued to report persistent feelings of loneliness. Although he enjoyed the volunteer's visits, he still felt left out, lacked a sense of belonging, and had difficulty engaging in activities that were meaningful for him. His sleep had become disrupted as one day blended into another, and he missed several key health appointments.

The psychiatrist learned of an intergenerational befriending program that took an individualized approach to target feelings of belonging and purpose for people who are homebound or otherwise having difficulty accessing group-based community interventions. After being referred, John received structured visits from two younger participants. Together, they collaborated with him on a creative project that brought him back to his college days as a theatre buff. At the end of the project, he had greater confidence about reengaging with others in the community, and he began reconnecting with some of his other retired workmates.

This psychiatrist recognized that every person experiencing loneliness is different. As a result, the effectiveness of community-based loneliness interventions varies from person to person. Customization and a personalized approach to every case is key to successful alleviation of loneliness. The availability of a variety of programs in the psychiatrist's and older man's community made it possible to tailor solutions for this patient.

Summary

Loneliness is a major public health issue that is increasingly recognized by governments, health insurers, health care professionals, communities, and citizens. COVID-19 has dispelled a common stereotype that loneliness is primarily a condition of older people, and this has helped refocus attention on the need to develop effective community interventions across the life span. Primary prevention measures must start early in schools to increase awareness of the importance of social connection for health and to short circuit the development of chronic loneliness in at-risk children and adolescents. Secondary prevention should focus on at-risk groups, such as those who are socially isolated or marginalized; those with mental, physical, and cognitive health conditions; caregivers; those who are bereaved; and those experiencing life transitions, such as geographical moves, school transitions, or retirement. In addition to cost-effective community interventions that recognize the needs of lonely people and those at risk, there is also a need for multilevel public policies that prioritize social health within populations to achieve the ultimate goal of creating "stable communities in which the terrible disease of loneliness can be cured."

KEY POINTS

- Governments across the world should focus their attention on addressing both the short- and long-term implications of loneliness and social isolation on health and quality of life as a public health priority.

- Greater attention must be paid to the evaluation and design of the built environment, social spaces, and social services to decrease loneliness and isolation as a matter of public policy and across sectors at the community, regional, and national levels.

- More methodologically strong research is needed to establish a comprehensive evidence base to inform effective public policies and community interventions for loneliness.

- Research is needed to understand the pathways by which socioeconomic disadvantage impacts loneliness and, reciprocally, how to address the health care and other economic costs of loneliness to individuals and societies.

Suggested Readings

Campaign to End Loneliness: campaigntoendloneliness.org

Donovan NJ, Blazer D: Social isolation and loneliness in older adults: review and commentary of a National Academies report. Am J Geriatr Psychiatry 28(12):1233–1244, 2020 32919873

Masi CM, Chen H-Y, Hawkley LC, Cacioppo JT: A meta-analysis of interventions to reduce loneliness. Pers Soc Psychol Rev 15(3):219–266, 2011 20716644

Poscia A, Stojanovic J, La Milia DI, et al: Interventions targeting loneliness and social isolation among the older people: an update systematic review. Exp Gerontol 102:133–144, 2018 29199121

Van Staden WC, Coetzee K: Conceptual relations between loneliness and culture. Curr Opin Psychiatry 23(6):524–529, 2010 20838346

References

Au A, Ng E, Garner B, et al: Proactive aging and intergenerational mentoring program to promote the well-being of older adults: pilot studies. Clin Gerontol 38(3):203–210, 2015

Bastoni S, Wrede C, Ammar A, et al: Psychosocial effects and use of communication technologies during home confinement in the first wave of the COVID-19 pandemic in Italy and the Netherlands. Int J Environ Res Public Health 18(5):2619, 2021 33807851

Bell P, Boissier N, Yaffe K, Lawlor B: P3-505: Multimodal Intergenerational Social Contact Intervention (MISCI). Alzheimer Dement 14(7S pt 24):P1315, 2018

Bell P, Allen IE, Jackson E, et al: P3-594: Feasibility, acceptability, and effectiveness of Multimodal Intergenerational Social Contact Intervention Pilot for Creative Engagement (MISCI-PCE) for older participants. Alzheimers Dement 15:1202, 2019

Bickerdike L, Booth A, Wilson PM, et al: Social prescribing: less rhetoric and more reality: a systematic review of the evidence. BMJ Open 7(4):e013384, 2017 28389486

Bolton M: Loneliness: The State We're In: A Report of Evidence Compiled for the Campaign to End Loneliness. Oxon, United Kingdom, Age UK Oxfordshire, 2012

Burns A, Leavey G, Ward M, et al: The impact of loneliness on healthcare use in older people: evidence from a nationally representative cohort. J Public Health 30:675–684, 2022

Carr DC, Kail BL, Matz-Costa C, Shavit YZ: Does becoming a volunteer attenuate loneliness among recently widowed older adults? J Gerontol B Psychol Sci Soc Sci 73(3):501–510, 2018 28977483

Casanova G, Zaccaria D, Rolandi E, Guaita A: The effect of information and communication technology and social networking site use on older people's well-being in relation to loneliness: review of experimental studies. J Med Internet Res 23(3):e23588, 2021 33439127

Cattan M, White M, Bond J, et al: Preventing social isolation and loneliness among older people: a systematic review of health promotion activities. Ageing Soc 25:41–67, 2005

Cattan M, Kime N, Bagnall AM: The use of telephone befriending in low level support for socially isolated older people: an evaluation. Health Soc Care Community 19(2):198–206, 2011 21114564

Centers for Disease Control and Prevention: Prioritizing Public Health Problems, Facilitator Guide. Atlanta, GA, Centers for Disease Control and Prevention, 2013

Czaja SJ, Boot WR, Charness N, et al: Improving social support for older adults through technology: findings from the PRISM randomized controlled trial. Gerontologist 58(3):467–477, 2018 28201730

Dickens AP, Richards SH, Greaves CJ, Campbell JL: Interventions targeting social isolation in older people: a systematic review. BMC Public Health 11(1):647, 2011, 21843337

Foster A, Thompson J, Holding E, et al: Impact of social prescribing to address loneliness: a mixed methods evaluation of a national social prescribing programme. Health Soc Care Community 29(5):1439–1449, 2021 33084083

Fried LP, Carlson MC, Freedman M, et al: A social model for health promotion for an aging population: initial evidence on the Experience Corps model. J Urban Health 81(1):64–78, 2004 15047786

Fried L, Prohaska T, Burholt V, et al: A unified approach to loneliness. Lancet 395(10218):114, 2020 31929010

Gaggioli A, Morganti L, Bonfiglio S, et al: Intergenerational group reminiscence: a potentially effective intervention to enhance elderly psychosocial wellbeing and to improve children's perception of aging. Educ Gerontol 40(7):486–498, 2014

Gerst-Emerson K, Jayawardhana J: Loneliness as a public health issue: the impact of loneliness on health care utilization among older adults. Am J Public Health 105(5):1013–1019, 2015 25790413

HM Government: A Connected Society: A Strategy for Tackling Loneliness: Laying the Foundations for Change. London, Department for Digital, Culture, Media and Sport, 2018

Holding E, Thompson J, Foster A, Haywood A: Connecting communities: a qualitative investigation of the challenges in delivering a national social prescribing service to reduce loneliness Health Soc Care Community 28(5):1535–1543, 2020 32166862

Jarrott SE, Turner SG, Naar JJ, et al: Increasing the power of intergenerational programs: Advancing an evaluation tool. J Appl Gerontol 41(3):763–768, 2022 34105401

Jetten J, Haslam SA, Cruwys T, et al: Advancing the social identity approach to health and well-being: progressing the social cure research agenda. Eur J Soc Psychol 47:789–802, 2017

Jopling K: Promising Approaches to Reducing Loneliness and Isolation in Later Life. London, Age UK, 2015

Jopling K, Sserwanja I: Loneliness Across the Life Course: A Rapid Review of the Evidence. Report. London, Calouste Gulbenkian Foundation, 2016

Kahlon MK, Aksan N, Aubrey R, et al: Effect of layperson-delivered, empathy-focused program of telephone calls on loneliness, depression, and anxiety among adults during the COVID-19 pandemic: a randomized clinical trial. JAMA Psychiatry 78(6):616–622, 2021

Kilgarriff-Foster A, O'Cathain A: Exploring the components and impact of social prescribing. J Public Ment Health 14(3):127–134, 2015

Kung CSJ, Kunz JS, Shields MA: Economic aspects of loneliness in Australia. Aust Econ Rev 54(1):147–163, 2021 34230671

Lai DWL, Li J, Ou X, et al: Effectiveness of a peer-based intervention on loneliness and social isolation of older Chinese immigrants in Canada: a randomized controlled trial. BMC Geriatr 20:356, 2020

Lawlor B, Golden J, Paul G, et al: Only the Lonely: A Randomized Controlled Trial of a Volunteer Visiting Programme for Older People Experiencing Loneliness. Technical Report. Dublin, Age Friendly Ireland, 2014

McDaid D, Bauer A, Park AL: Making the Economic Case for Investing in Actions to Prevent and/or Tackle Loneliness: A Systematic Review. London, LSE, 2017

McHugh JE, Kenny RA, Lawlor BA, et al: The discrepancy between social isolation and loneliness as a clinically meaningful metric: findings from the Irish and English longitudinal studies of ageing (TILDA and ELSA). Int J Geriatr Psychiatry 32(6):664–674, 2017

Michaelson J, Jeffrey K, Abdallah S: The cost of loneliness to UK employers: the impact of loneliness upon business across the UK. London, New Economics Foundation, February 20, 2017

National Academies of Sciences, Engineering, and Medicine: Social Isolation and Loneliness in Older Adults: Opportunities for the Health Care System. Washington, DC, The National Academies Press, 2020

National Health Service: The NHS Long Term Plan. London, National Health Service, 2019. Available at: www.longtermplan.nhs.uk/wp-content/uploads/2019/08/nhs-long-term-plan-version-1.2.pdf.

New Economics Foundation and The Co-Op. Report 2017

Noone C, McSharry J, Smalle M, et al: Video calls for reducing social isolation and loneliness in older people: a rapid review. Cochrane Database Syst Rev 5(5):CD013632, 2020 32441330

O'Luanaigh CO, Lawlor BA: Loneliness and the health of older people. Int J Geriatr Psychiatry 23(12):1213–1221, 2008 18537197

Polley MJ, Bertotti M, Kimberlee R, et al: A Review of the Evidence Assessing Impact of Social Prescribing on Healthcare Demand and Cost Implications. Westminster, United Kingdom, University of Westminster, 2017

Prohaska T, Burholt V, Burns A, et al: Consensus statement: loneliness in older adults, the 21st century social determinant of health? BMJ Open 10(8):e034967, 2020

Suzuki K, Dollery BE, Kortt MA: Addressing loneliness and social isolation amongst elderly people through local co-production in Japan. Soc Policy Adm 55(4):674–686, 2021

Valtorta NK, Kanaan M, Gilbody S, et al: Loneliness, social isolation and social relationships: what are we measuring? A novel framework for classifying and comparing tools. BMJ Open 6:e010799, 2016

Vonnegut K: Palm Sunday: An Autobiographical Collage. New York, Delacorte, 1981

Williams CYK, Townson AT, Kapur M, et al: Interventions to reduce social isolation and loneliness during COVID-19 physical distancing measures: a rapid systematic review. PLoS One 16(2):e0247139, 2021 33596273

Index

Page numbers printed in **boldface** type refer to tables and figures.